"WHAT TO KNOW . . .

WHEN *SHE'S* EXPECTING"

A survival guide for fathers

** Cover by Donna Watts*

WE WANT TO HEAR FROM YOU!

If you have any suggestions that you feel might enhance the contents of this book, please send them to:

Blue Shoes Publishing, Inc.
P.O. Box 20968
Louisville Ky. 40220

Unfortunately, we cannot send payment for your suggestions. We are simply too cheap. However, if your suggestions are accepted, then you will be helping other fathers who may benefit from your insight.

SECOND PRINTING

Library of Congress Cataloging - in - Publication Data

Bays, Harold 1958

"What to Know When She's Expecting"

Library of Congress Catalog Card Number: 97-093295
Soft-cover Trade ISBN: 0-9647944-3-8

DEDICATION

This book is dedicated to all the men who have repeatedly been told how they should be more "involved" in the whole pregnancy situation, only to find that, after making their biological contribution, "involvement" really means doing what ***she*** says.

SPECIAL THANKS

The authors wish to thank their wives, who should be given due credit for their participation in the whole pregnancy situation.

DISCLAIMER

Nothing in this book should be taken too seriously. These are only the opinions of the authors. Always check with the experts before making any decisions regarding the whole pregnancy situation.

And if her family is not available, you might check with the doctor.

(***Note:*** At least one of the wives of the authors agrees that ***certain*** men can often be insensitive during the whole pregnancy situation. However, she would like it known that the suggestion that women may be emotional or irrational during this period has no relevance to her own pregnancy situation. She, frankly, has no idea what the book is talking about.)

FETAL DEVELOPMENT CHART

Day 0: One of your sperm has penetrated her egg to create a complete, one-celled, first stage embryo called a zygote.

Day 6: The zygote has undergone multiple divisions, and the multi celled embryo implants into the womb (uterus).

Week 3: The embryo's heart begins to beat. Upper limbs, eyes, and ears begin to form.

Week 4: The lower limbs and eyes are beginning to form.

Week 8: The beginnings of all essential structures are present. The eyes are closed, the head is enlarged, and the ears are low set. The sex organs are not distinguishable yet as to male or female.

Week 15: Fingernail development has occurred for about the past five weeks. Now toenails are beginning to develop.

Week 20: The head and body hair are visible. The mother may have begun feeling movements of the fetus. Ultrasound can probably determine the gender of the fetus.

Week 22: The fetus could potentially survive outside the womb.

Week 30: The fetus now has fingernails, toenails, eyelashes, good head of hair, and eyes that are wide open.

Week 40: The baby is due.

A SPECIAL NOTE TO THE "POLITICALLY CORRECT"

Now that we are in our second printing, we are pleased that most of our most avid readers and supporters have been ***women.*** Because, unless read with the most superficial and defensive mind-set, most open-minded women have found "What to Know" a humorous, educational tool that encourages the man to be more active in the whole pregnancy situation by improving ***his*** knowledge, and by acknowledging ***his*** perspective, in a format that he might actually read.

But this woman support comes as no surprise. Because the content of this book was derived, not only from the personal experiences of the authors, but from many meetings with women, who gave us their best "men and pregnancy" stories. So, while not all aspects of this book may apply to all couples, it does reflect the realities of many pregnancies - as documented by women.

The point is, most women genuinely care about what the man is experiencing during an event in which all attention is usually directed only towards the woman. The irony has been that, at the same time that men are being encouraged to play a more active role in the whole pregnancy situation, many of ***their*** issues (such as those raised in this book) are too often dismissed, or flat out ignored. Therefore, for those women who really do care about what the man might actually be experiencing during this ***mutual*** event, then, as we see it, they have one of three options: (1) just ask him about his feelings - and we all know how fruitful that conversation might be, (2) read books discussing how men are suppose to feel - probably written by women, or (3) read ***this*** book.

Because, this book is not just humor, it is not just stereotyped rhetoric, but in many realities, it is simply the truth.

CONTENTS

Chapter 1: Is she pregnant?

"The bottom-line is that pregnancy is always associated with a loss of the menstrual period, unless it isn't, and a missed menstrual period always means pregnancy, unless it is due to something else."

Question: *She normally hates to cook. But today, she called me at work to tell me that she had some news, and that she wanted to cook me a very special supper. Could she be pregnant?*

Answer: No question about it. On the other hand, she may have wrecked the car, or just invited her parents to stay for a week.

Question: *Upon arriving home, I noticed small socks taped to the mantle. When I asked what they were, she called them "booties." What are "booties," and what are they doing on the mantle? Did Christmas come early? Now, she's looking at me really weird, like I should know what she is trying to tell me. But I am a man. What do I do?*

Answer: You better check your schedule - for about the next eighteen years.

Question: *We have been sexually active. We have not used birth control. In the past few months, she has missed her menstrual periods, has been hungry all day, has been sick every morning, and has been urinating all the time. Could she be pregnant?*

Answer: Two possibilities may exist. First of all, she may have simply misplaced her uterus, thus causing her to miss her menstrual period. In her anxiety and confusion over this loss, she may have resorted to eating odd foods such as ice cream and pickles, thus causing sickness in the morning, with extension of this sickness onto the bladder, resulting in the need to urinate all the time.

Or . . . she could be pregnant.

Question: *She is normally a very light sleeper. Yesterday, a tornado took the roof off our house. She never woke up. Could she be pregnant?*

Answer: Yes.

Question: *She normally loves pepperoni pizza with onions. Last night, I mentioned that I had this for lunch at work. She threw up all over the bathroom. Could she be pregnant?*

Answer: You bet.

Question: *When she got done with writing a letter, she stood up and suddenly became very lightheaded. After I grabbed her to prevent her fall, she said that her breasts were so painful, that they were killing her. She then began to cry. When I asked why, she said she felt so sad for Bambi. I have no idea what she's talking about. Could she be pregnant?*

Answer: Absolutely.

Question: *We have been dating, and have been sexually active. Although she has never considered this a serious relationship, she just asked me for a wedding ring. Could she be pregnant?*

Answer: Better brush off the tux, big boy.

Question: *She just gave me this book as a gift. Could she be pregnant?*

Answer: Probably, unless she has a really odd sense of humor. In that case, she may or may not be pregnant.

Question: *She missed her last menstrual period, but has no other symptoms or signs of pregnancy. Could she be pregnant?*

Answer: The signs and symptoms of pregnancy are variable among women, and many times, nonspecific. For example, some women can exhibit signs of pregnancy, only to find that they are suffering from the ill-effects of an unkind helping of lasagna, or perhaps, the betrayal of her previous friends, Jim Beam and Jack Daniels.

On the other hand, we've all heard the stories on the news about some woman who had no idea she was pregnant until she felt her water break at the mall or something.

Therefore, it is essential that a basic concept be made crystal clear.

The most common cause of a missed menstrual period in a woman of childbearing potential (who otherwise has normal menstrual periods) is always pregnancy. This is a universal law, with only two exceptions. First of all, she may become pregnant and still have a subsequent light, or even normal menstrual period afterward. Secondly, a missed menstrual period can occur during periods of fatigue, stress, fear, poor nutrition, heavy exercise, weight loss or weight gain, medical illnesses, and/or stopping of birth control pills.

The bottom-line is that pregnancy is always associated with a loss of the menstrual period, unless it isn't, and a missed menstrual period always means pregnancy, unless it is due to something else.

Hopefully, this clarifies this very important issue.

Question: *She has not had a menstrual period in months. Her mother told her to get a pregnancy test. But since we have not used birth control for more than two years, and since she has not gotten pregnant in the past, I know she* ***can't*** *be pregnant now. My mother-in-law is clearly neurotic. But what else could be the problem?*

Answer: The main problem is that you don't seem to have a clue what's going on. Just because you went more than two years without birth control, and without a pregnancy, mean absolutely nothing. Unless you or she has a fertility problem, it is a good bet that if you can supply the seed, she can probably grow it. Finally, you better straighten-up that attitude regarding your mother-in-law. Stay on her good side, and she will make your life much easier. Get on her bad side, and you may soon find that . . . well . . . let's just say that in a relative sense, you might find times when you actually look forward to dental work.

Question: *It is conceivable she might be pregnant. Now what do we do?*

Answer: First of all, the use of the word "conceivable" was a nice touch. In response to your question, the answer is simple: get a pregnancy test. Go ahead. Get involved. Try six or eight of 'em. They're relatively inexpensive. They're really a blast. And you'll be conducting highly important scientific testing. You'll feel like you're back in eighth grade chemistry, only without the Bunsen burners.

You will become, in essence, Mr. Science.

It's your choice. So enjoy it because it may be the last choice you have for many years to come.

CHAPTER 1: Is she pregnant?

Question: *We have tried to conceive a baby for over a year. Recently, my wife stated that an over-the-counter pregnancy test was positive. Is it possible that she may have a hormone-secreting tumor? Could she have drunk something that reacted with the test? I understand that cows are injected with hormones. She had beef last night. Could this have caused the positive urine test?*

Answer: Tumors of the adrenal gland and ovary can rarely produce hormones that can cross react with pregnancy urine tests. They are incredibly rare. It is doubtful that she could have drunk anything that caused a reaction with the home pregnancy test. Some cows are injected with bovine somatotropin, which makes them bigger. But this has nothing to do with urine pregnancy tests.

And finally, she is pregnant.

Question: *The results of our pregnancy test are positive. Do we still need to go see a doctor?*

Answer: Most home urine pregnancy tests measure for hCG, which stands for human chorionic gonadotropin (we knew you were dying to know). An antibody in the test kit reacts with this hormone to cause a chemical reaction that changes the indicator color, as well as the rest of your life.

These tests are most accurate about 10 days after conception. In fact, if the test is positive, and she is not receiving certain unusual hormone drugs, there is more than a 95% chance she is pregnant.

If the test is negative, then five main possibilities exist:

(1) She is not pregnant.

(2) She did not wait long enough before doing the test. (Most experts recommend waiting a few days after the missed menstrual period.)

(3) She has an ectopic pregnancy that can sometimes be harder to detect.

(4) She didn't urinate on the stick correctly. (We don't know how that's possible either.)

(5) The test is defective or outdated. (And if you have so many urine pregnancy test kits that some have become outdated, then you are just way too involved in this whole pregnancy testing situation.)

Most home pregnancy tests tell you in the instructions to always follow-up any positive results with the doctor, who may then perform a pregnancy blood test that is not terribly more accurate, but may cost a whole lot more. So congratulate yourself for helping our health care industry grow and prosper.

In any event, while the ***urine*** pregnancy test is accurate more than 95% of the time, the ***blood*** pregnancy test is accurate more than 99% of the time.

If you need to sit in the waiting room of the OB/GYN's office until the blood test is complete, make sure you take a good look around. There's a good chance that you'll be spending a lot of time sitting in this very room looking at a lot of pregnant women. It can sometimes be overwhelming. Also, you may notice the "interesting" reading material such as a 1979 issue of Home Journal.

And if the OB/GYN doctor happens to be a woman, you may notice other magazines with fascinating articles like:

"Ten Ways to Change Him Into What You Want Him to Be,"

or

"How to Tell Him About His Insensitivity, and His Other Faults"

or

"Why Men Think You Want to Change Them, and Why They Think You're Such a Nag."

You may also note the shortage of "Sports Illustrated." So bring a book - any book.

Bring this book.

Once you receive the results of the OB/GYN's test, the games may officially begin. It's going to be a stressful and bizarre time no matter what happens. So stay calm and try to retain your sense of humor. Bring a ferret with you to the OB/GYN's office and let it run around the waiting room. Or, loudly eat an entire bag of potato chips for every 15 minutes you have to wait.

The office staff may get upset. But you should get a good laugh out of it.

And besides, you're a man, so they should know what to expect.

Chapter 2: What to know, now that she's pregnant

"Now that she is expecting, your feelings are irrelevant. Your commitments are irrelevant. Your sacrifices are irrelevant. Now that she is expecting, you are relevant only in how well you understand that you can never understand what she is going through."

Life Changes

Question: *One of the reasons she chose me as her partner is because I am an outgoing person with many hobbies. I love my work, and work all the time. I love sports, TV remote controls, and partying with my friends. And I literally can spend days on my computer, surfing the Internet, and trying to figure out the latest computer software. Now that she's expecting, is any of this going to change?*

Answer: Yes.

In the mystical past, fathers (reportedly) were minimally involved in the day-to-day care of children. Men would hunt, provide food/ protection, and otherwise be engaged in manly things. Women would breast feed, and manage the home (cave, house, whatever). However, many women are now as involved in their careers as men - if not more. And in many families, two incomes are needed, just to make ends meet. Therefore, the social mind-set has changed. Men are now expected to play a more active role, starting at conception.

Nevertheless, even today, it is occasionally reported that some men still choose to distance themselves from the whole pregnancy situation (hey, it's your prerogative, Mr. Cro-Magnon). And to those who are considering running away (figuratively, or literally), you need to quit being such a coward, and face the challenge with the rest of us - and stop being such a spineless weenie.

In other words, if you feel that your lifestyle will somehow be threatened by the presence of a child, then you are absolutely right. Yes, you may feel resentment about these changes. And this resentment could manifest itself through nastiness to her, or to your child, causing the poor kid to turn out to be a notorious mobster, or a certain shameless political figure.

So you need to get a grip on the reality of the situation. Life, as you know it, is over.

Question: *For years, I have liked to hang out with friends at a local bar down the street. I first met her there. After we started dating, I quit going as much. When we got married, I only went there about twice a week. Now that she's pregnant, I only go about once a week, by myself. But even so, she seems upset whenever I go. She tells me that with the new baby coming, I have other responsibilities now.*

I don't have anything left that defines me as an individual. Our house is ours, our possessions are ours, and on the rare occasions when we do go out, we go out together. This bar is the only place left where I can go and just be myself. At the bar with my friends, I am not a husband, a father, or a job title.

I am just me.

After the whole pregnancy situation is over, will she let me go back to my one last refuge as an individual, even if it is just once every other week?

Answer: No.

Question: *Before she was expecting, we had a relationship, based on mutual considerations of each other feelings. We tried to understand each other's commitments to such things as career. And we always expressed how much we appreciated each other's sacrifices. But now that she is expecting, things seem to have changed? Why?*

Answer: Now that she is expecting, your feelings are irrelevant. Your commitments are irrelevant. Your sacrifices are irrelevant. Now that she is expecting, you are relevant only in how well you understand that you can never understand what she is going through.

Question*: How do I handle changes in my life, now that she is expecting?*

Answer: Try to rationalize. Tell yourself that this pregnancy portends a new challenge and a time of amazing discovery. This experience is simply an opportunity to expand the parameters of your lifestyle, and any sacrifice you make now will be returned to you tenfold down the line. You are engaged in a training session of the ages that will prepare you to manage, mold, and influence the most ultimate of miracles, currently manifest in the most helpless of creatures. You are standing at the precipice of your existence, peering at the cavernous void that will soon become filled with the most perfect creation in the known universe.

If that doesn't work, just whine and complain a lot. But understand that no one really cares. After all, ***she's*** the one who's expecting.

Conflicting Attitudes

Question: *She knew that I did not want another child. However, she stopped her birth control pills on her own (without letting me know), and now she is pregnant. I am really angry, frustrated, and resentful. What do I do?*

Answer: First of all, you have every right to be angry, frustrated, and resentful. And what she did was wrong. No one parent should have the final say as to whether or not a new life is to be brought into the world. This has to be a mutual decision.

So what do you do? Basically, you're stuck with few options. Clearly, you probably understand that, no matter what happened, the child is not the one who should pay the price.

So the real issue is, what do you do with her?

First of all, you could do exactly what she (and probably her family and friends) thinks you should do. You could give in, and forgive and forget. You could simply forgive, and otherwise accept the situation with a loving attitude. And you could simply forget her actions without ever feeling a sense of utter betrayal. And if you can do these things, then God Bless you. Because you are a better man than most.

Secondly, you could forgive, but not forget. In other words, you could accept your responsibility as a new father, regardless of the circumstances. And you could continue to love her, despite what she has done. But in the back of your mind, you know that you will always remember.

Finally, you could neither forgive nor forget. In this case, you may be tempted to leave her, and/or the child. If this option seems quite reasonable, or likely, then obtain counsel first. Don't make a mistake you may regret, regardless of what she has done.

Question: *I am really excited that she is expecting, because I really wanted another child. But I'm not sure she did. And now that she is pregnant, I don't think she is all that excited. This worries me because if something goes wrong during the pregnancy, I feel like it will be my fault. What do I do?*

Answer: No one parent should have the final say as to whether or not a new life is to be brought into the world. This has to be a mutual decision. And if you essentially forced the whole pregnancy situation, then you may be headed for problems with your relationship with her. If so, you might try talking to her about your feelings and fears, or recommend that you and she seek counseling.

With regard to the pregnancy, neither parent should feel guilty if something goes wrong as the result of chance. Even if all precautions are taken, and everything is done exactly right, it is simply a statistical fact that a certain number of pregnancies will result in problems such as a miscarriage, or a congenital/chromosomal abnormality. You may wonder why you may have been so unlucky, but you should never blame yourself, or her. As hard as it may be to accept, some things are just nobody's fault.

Think of it this way, are you your parents' fault?

Chapter 3: What to know throughout her pregnancy

"This is natural. It is not normal."

Mood Swings and Behavior

Question: *Since she's been expecting, I've noticed that she seems to be moody and irrational at times. Is this common?*

Answer: Really? Moody ***and*** irrational? This question required a thorough search in the reference vault, the Index Medicus, as well as the Alta Vista search engine on the Internet. Sure enough, apparently moodiness and irrational behavior are sometimes associated with pregnancy.

Fascinating.

Question: *Since she's been expecting, I've noticed that she seems to be moody and irrational at times. Is this natural? Is this normal?*

Answer: In nature, it is a rare, but natural occurrence that an otherwise content and normal star can suddenly explode without warning, resulting in a supernova outburst of destructive energy. At the peak of this event, the explosion can outshine an entire galaxy. Afterward, a surrounding radioactive cloud may form, resulting in harmful remnants that persist long after the initial explosion.

This is natural. It is not normal.

Question: *I have heard that once she's expecting, she may become moody and irrational at times. Why?*

Answer: Some women actually become calmer, and less stressed during pregnancy. They may find that matters that used to be so important in the past, take a second seat to the awesome prospect of carrying an unborn child. In these cases, stress reactions such as stomach upset, sleeplessness, and anger may actually improve.

But don't count on it.

If mood swings and irrational behavior occur, they may seem most intense during the first trimester, when hormonal cocktails are being mixed and served for your pleasure. If this occurs, you may find yourself at times drowning in a sea of estrogen, and being pummeled by wave after wave of crashing emotional tides. And try as you will to stop the flood, it is the natural law of our times that you receive the brunt of the impact. Because regardless of the real, or perceived problem, it ***will*** be your fault.

From a practical standpoint, you need to be prepared to find yourself shocked (and maybe a little afraid) of your once docile and loving companion, who may suddenly change into a seething, fire-spitting she-beast, only to just as suddenly change back into the woman you knew - as though nothing ever happened.

This is natural. It is not normal.

Question: *We just found out last week that she's expecting. I have tried to be sensitive to her needs. But today, I thoughtlessly made a peanut butter sandwich, using the "crunchy" instead of the "smooth" jar. (I don't know what I was thinking).*

Understandably, she screamed, shrieked, screeched, howled, wailed, moaned, sobbed, wept, whimpered, whined and otherwise made it clear she was upset. She then threw the peanut butter jar through the window and began smashing dishes in an attempt to compromise the very foundation of the house. She became so angry that she told me to "get out of my sight!" But when I left, she asked "Where are you going?"

What did this mean? How should I have responded?

Answer: When she is expecting, it is natural (it is not normal) for her to say such things. It is therefore essential that you develop a sensitivity toward understanding, not what she ***says***, but what she really ***means.*** For example, when she said "get out of my sight," she may have really meant one of three things.

First of all, she may have meant that she was feeling bad, and simply wanted a hug.

Secondly, it is equally likely that she really wanted you to get out of her sight.

But thirdly, it is also possible that she wanted a hug, ***and*** she wanted you to get out of her sight.

So how should you have responded?

We have no idea.

But you might try this. Treat the whole situation like you are living in a bizarre mystery thriller, where you never know who may be lurking around the next corner. Be prepared to adapt to any situation. Make it a challenge to be on your toes at all times. Expect the unexpected. On page one, you might be sharing an innocent moment with the girl of your dreams. But as quickly as you turn the page, she might suddenly change into a nightmare behemoth waiting to suck all the blood out of your uncaring, inconsiderate, thoughtless little veins.

You need to be careful out there.

Question: *Since she's been expecting, she has recurring nightmares about me being with other women. Why?*

Answer: In survey after survey, the number one concern of women is not balancing the federal budget, is not job security, is not professional and financial success, and is not even the win/loss record of your local sports team. (Hard to believe.) As foreign as it may be to you, the number one concern of most women is: low self esteem.

And apparently, as she evolves into a cannon ball-carrying bag of hormones, she thinks of herself as less attractive, and less desirable.

Furthermore, she is now face-to-face with the knowledge that she will soon have the primary responsibility of sacrificing and providing for another demanding, totally dependent, helpless human being (other than you).

And knowing that she can rarely trust you to even take out the garbage, it is probably not unreasonable for her to worry about your ability and willingness to accept your role as a responsible adult and father.

By the way, when ***was*** the last time you took out the trash?

Question: *Since she's been expecting, she has gotten a lot more religious. Is this natural? Is this normal?*

Answer: Many women find that being involved in the whole life-creation situation is a spiritual experience. And considering all the potential risks and rewards, and all the certainties and uncertainties, it is no surprise that she may become overwhelmed and seek comfort and guidance from a greater power.

Add to this all the known and unforeseen financial bills that lie ahead, and both of you can use all the help you can get.

This is both natural, and very normal.

Family

Question*: It seems like now that she's pregnant, my in-laws are around a lot more, offering lots of advice that I don't always agree with. Do I have to be nice to them?*

Answer: When she is expecting, you will most likely intensify your relationship with your in-laws, and your own parents. This can be a problem. For example, although they may never have spoken, it will seem, at times, as if everyone had a telepathic conference in the car on the way over, and decided that everything you've ever said, done, or thought was wrong. Therefore, it is essential that you respectfully, but forcibly, put your foot down as soon as possible to establish who's really the boss, and that everyone needs to shut up and do what ***she*** says.

The thing is, it is likely that they've been through it. The other thing is, it is likely that a lot has changed. So, although much of their advice is valuable, some of it may be garbage. Therefore, you will have to learn how to agree that they are probably right much of the time. But you should emphasize that, occasionally, you may have to defer to current medical science, and may even have to follow the advice of the doctor, even if it conflicts with Grandma's collection of "words of ultimate gestational wisdom."

Question: *I had a really good relationship with my father when I was growing up. Now that she's expecting, I wonder how my relationship with my child will compare with my relationship with my father?*

Answer: The relationship between you and your dad was, is, and will always be a separate entity. However, now may be a good time to plan how you can apply those valuable lessons you learned from your father. For example, you should try to remember all his instructive stories that were to somehow positively influence your life. Who can forget how, "when he was a child," he walked mile after mile through the frozen snow to go to school. And what about how he gave up his promising business/sports/music/modeling/etc. (pick one) career, just because of you. Although it may seem unclear how any of these stories provide any useful benefit toward the successful upbringing of a child, they are nonetheless, a time-honored tradition. Therefore, you should start making up equally as ridiculous, irrelevant, overblown, and self-serving anecdotes today, so that you are prepared in the near future.

Question: *I always fought with my father when I was growing up. We continue to fight today. Now that she's expecting, I wonder how my relationship with my child will compare with my relationship with my father?*

Answer: As noted before, the relationship between you and your dad was, is, and will always be a separate entity. If you and your dad constantly fight, now may be a good time to try and improve things. You may find that your dad goes nuts over the prospect of your new baby, even while your relationship could be better. You may even eventually find that he is better able to communicate with your child, than he does with you. This may be because you both have unresolved feelings that you are unable to communicate, or because in your child he sees an unspoiled version of you.

Or it could simply be because your kid is a better listener than you were, are, or ever will be.

CHAPTER 3: Throughout her pregnancy

Question: *My dad left my mom and me when I was a child. I have rarely, if ever, seen him since. Although I still have some resentment and anger, I mostly just don't care. As far as I am concerned, I have no father. Now that she is expecting, do I have to let him know he is a grandfather?*

Answer: Forget him. If he abandoned you and your mother simply because he had other things to do, he is not worth your time. If you still have some unresolved issues that bother you, then send him a postcard with a quick note of "by the way, we had a kid." With regard to which postcard might be most appropriate, you might try one that sports "Wish You Were Here," and hand write below "yeah, for about the past two decades."

He probably won't care. But you might get a good laugh out of it.

Question: *Friends of ours have told us that once you have a baby, you start neglecting your pets. I have a very special relationship with our dog. Is my dog going to suffer?*

Answer: Neglect is certainly a strong word for it, but yes, your relationships with your pets are probably going to change - unless your pet is a goldfish. In this case, simply feeding and cleaning are all that is required, and chances are, the necessity of sharing affections probably won't matter much.

Goldfish are a lot like men in that way.

Cats become accustomed to a certain lifestyle, and are definitely going to notice some differences. Many couples promise their cats that everything will be the same as it ever was once the baby comes. And it is so tragic when they are proven wrong.

Dogs are quite adaptable. But even they need reassurance that they will continue to be at least one of your best friends.

So while your partner is pregnant, pay as much attention to your animal friends as you possibly can. You may want to try to prepare your pet for what is approaching. If you know someone who has a small baby, invite them over and use their child as an experiment to see how your pet reacts. (Why risk your own kid?) If they get along, great! If they don't, threaten your dog with a trip to the veterinarian where he may get that special kind of operation that the neighbor's dog had. You know, the kind of operation where afterward, Butch just sits around the house and stares at everyone with that "why am I alive" look.

Once the baby comes, your pet will most likely recondition itself to accommodate the new arrival. And eventually, both of them may even become buddies, forging an alliance so that they can plan a strategic move against you in the future.

Money

Question: *I am concerned about money now that she is expecting. Because our health insurance agent, "Bob," always cared so deeply about us as human beings, he always made sure* *that we had the best health insurance coverage, no matter how high the premium. Considering that we have faithfully paid our health insurance premiums for years, now that she is expecting, can we expect that we will receive premium medical treatment.*

Answer: Questions such as this tax the very boundaries of reality.

Yes, once upon a time, doctors made the sole decisions as to what was in the best medical interest of their patients. Unfortunately, too many doctors (and their patients) abused this privilege, and thus abused the system. Hospitalizations would be inappropriately used for things like simple physical exams because "it would be more convenient to get everything done in the hospital." The doctor and hospital would then send outrageous bills for these dubious admissions to the health insurance companies.

As a result, most insurance companies now direct a substantial amount of what and where health care ***is*** provided, and what and where care ***is not*** provided. For example, as hard as it may be to believe, doctors used to determine the most appropriate length of time patients stayed in the hospital, the most appropriate medicines prescribed, and the most appropriate procedure for the individual patient based upon what was in the best interest of the patient.

Hard to believe.

Now many health insurance companies now release doctors from the need to make such difficult decisions.

So if you have concerns that you may not receive the level of health care you expected while she's expecting, due to problems with insurance coverage, then contact your agent "Bob." Because of your past, wonderful and caring relationship with him, ask him to be your advocate in persuading the insurance company to allow her a few extra hours in the hospital to recover, if the doctor thinks it is best, after she delivers.

You probably won't get anywhere. But he should get a good laugh out of it.

But before you get all mad and crazy at the whole insurance situation, ask yourself this:

> *In an otherwise normal pregnancy situation, when and how did giving birth become an "illness" that warrants health insurance coverage?*

If you answer this honestly, you may be more inclined to allow the insurance company some slack.

Question: *Now that she's expecting, she wants me to keep up with the medical bills. But I keep getting bill after bill from the insurance company that states "This Is Not a Bill." At the same time, I also get bill after bill from the doctor and hospital indicating that I really do have a bill. What is going on?*

Answer: Doctors and hospitals make money by receiving payment of bills. And with shrinking health care dollars, they want the cash - NOW! But sometimes the billing process is so confusing, that it is almost impossible to know what you really owe, even if you wanted to send a check to those underpaid doctors and hospitals. And insurance companies often don't make it any easier by sending statements that list charges of services, but then also note that the statement is "Not a Bill." Although it is far less than clear, apparently, these "Not a Bill" documents (only understood by CPA's, or IRS agents), are simply to "inform" the patient about what has been paid, what will be covered, and/or what won't be covered.

And while you are mired in trying to figure out what is, and what is not a bill, the doctor and hospital become increasingly impatient about nonpayment, with the end result that you get sent to a collection agency because you did not pay a statement that was "Not a Bill."

A good rule of thumb is that if you have already met your deductible, and you receive a bill from the hospital or doctor, then you probably should pay it. If you have any questions about whether or not you really received the services listed on the bill, then contact the friendly billing personnel at the hospital or doctor's office. They are always a cheery group that are just too happy to deal with inquisitive people like you.

Alternatively, if you feel that the insurance company has made a mistake, then just call them. But have a copy of your "Not a Bill" close by, so that you will have documentation to intelligently discuss the problem.

Finally, the best number to call the insurance company is probably a 1-800 number. Just be sure to block off the afternoon so you have plenty of time to enjoy hours of great phone music, as you wait for them to answer the call. And don't worry if you are confused about the whole "Not a Bill" situation, because you will probably find the insurance billing personnel as friendly, and as helpful as those at the hospital or doctor's office.

Propaganda and record keeping

Question: *Every time she goes to the doctor, and every time she goes to the hospital for tests, she always brings back brochures with a section for the father. Also, she is constantly getting newsletters that also have a "section for fathers." Who comes up with this stuff? Who has time to read this stuff? I know she is going to ask me if I read them. What do I do?*

Answer: These sections for "for the father" are actually wish-list propaganda written by women, for women. Their intent is to point out deficiencies that you have, or will soon develop, simply because you are a man. From a practical standpoint, you will receive mounds of this material. You will be expected to read it. You won't. She will ask you to answer questions about it. You won't. And the next several days of your life will be an examination of your insensitivity.

Therefore, you must memorize the following:

"Well honey, I believe the article correctly pointed out

what an emotional time this is for you, and how I need to be more understanding."

If you know this one line, you will probably be accurate 90% of the time. And even if you are totally off, it will likely be a better answer than if you had actually read the articles.

***Question**: I'm interested in keeping a "Baby Journal." How do I start?*

Answer: A "Baby Journal" is an excellent idea for expectant fathers. It will allow you to express your feelings during this amazing time in your life. And as long as you don't let anyone know, it may be one of the only chances you have of making your own decision during the whole pregnancy situation.

If you have a computer, just get a word-processing program, and start writing. You can save the journal for as long as you'd like, or secretly print it out to bore others. Certain programs will also allow you to add flourishes to your journal, using interesting type fonts, illustrations or page decorations. Use your imagination; there are certainly no rules when it comes to this kind of project.

Blank journal books are available at book stores and office supply stores. The problem is that it is unlikely that these journal books will have masculine covers. Instead, they will probably have ornately decorated covers, making you feel compelled to explain to the check out clerk why you - as a man - are purchasing such a thing. Therefore, you need to have some good sports stories on hand, or be ready to explain that you couldn't find any journals with the pictures of wrestlers on the cover. Alternatively, you may just roll your eyes and sheepishly admit you liked the cover, and hope your fellow man understands.

He probably won't. But he should get a good laugh out of it.

(As an alternative to the flower-covered journal, you might consider getting a black business journal. Although this may seem like an odd choice for recording baby stuff, you will at least have preserved some of your manhood).

Regardless of what journal you choose, the words in this journal will be handwritten, which will add sentimentality to the journal and make it a little more personal. It does not, sadly, offer a "spell check." Therefore, if you ever decide to give it to your child at a later date, you will have documented your inability of mastering the English language.

But since you are a man, it probably won't make that much difference to your reputation.

Once you have decided what form the journal will be in, the next logical step will be to figure out what you're going to write. This will be easy for some, and difficult for others. The important thing is to be sincere; you are writing this journal for your baby. And these words will be a part of the child's life for a long time to come. In an attempt to increase the chances that your child may have an interest in reading this later on, you may wish to address your journal entries directly to the baby, such as:

CHAPTER 3: Throughout her pregnancy

"You are growing bigger in your mother's belly."

If you child ends up being a girl, she will enjoy this very much. She will think it was very "sweet." If your child ends up being a boy, he'll just think you were a little weird. But his wife might enjoy it very much.

So you might approach this as a kind of a diary, meant not so much for the baby, but more for yourself. After all, it will probably be cheaper than therapy. Every day of the pregnancy can be a revelation if you choose to look at it that way. Getting in touch and communicating your feelings may prove to be a rewarding experience. Conversely, it may also be a visit to the worst hell ever imagined. After all, how many pages can be dedicated to:

"Day 272. She is still expecting. I have nothing else to say."

The point is, not every man has the ability or desire to write what they are feeling. And not every man has any particular feelings at all times. So if you are an "emotionally challenged" man, don't worry. Just go to the book store and find a book of what you probably should be feeling, and writing, as a man. (The book will probably have been written by a woman.) This may be more your speed, and may prove more fulfilling to your child, once he or she is old enough to care about it.

Sex

Question: *Can we have sex, now that she's expecting?*

Answer: Hey, it's your prerogative Mr. Cro-Magnon.

But first of all, at various points during the whole pregnancy situation, she may look and feel like her uterus is housing a watermelon. She may have sleepiness, fatigue, nausea, indigestion, and have the need to urinate all the time. She may also have acne, colored stretch marks on her belly, varicose veins, constipation, nasal congestion, nosebleeds, bleeding gums, back pain, leg cramps, leg swelling, hemorrhoids, shortness of breath, false labor pains, loss of balance, nipple drainage, a navel that is about to explode, and pain in the pelvis and buttocks region.

The point is, she may not feel pretty.

But although some women may have a decreased interest in sex during pregnancy, other women actually enjoy sex better. So, for her sake, feel free to ask (beg) frequently.

Secondly, intercourse during the last few months may result in you hitting the uterus covering the baby's head. If this happens, it is unlikely that you are going to cause any damage to the baby's skull. (No matter how much you think of yourself, you are just not that much of a man). However, most doctors recommend that if you do run the risk of hitting the baby's head, it's time to stop. Because, if for no other reason, it seems like a really rude thing to do.

Thirdly, certain circumstances may exist in which sexual intercourse should be restricted during pregnancy, such as if she has unexplained vaginal bleeding, if she has a history of miscarriages, or if she has "placenta previa." Also, intercourse should not occur during the last trimester if she has a history of premature labor, or if she expecting more than one child (i.e., twins etc.).

Also, if she has broken her water, or is in active labor, it is probably best to prioritize your efforts towards preparing for delivery. Insisting on sex during active labor will only encourage her, and her family and friends, to tag you with that ill-deserved "insensitive," and "selfish" label again.

Finally, it is important that someone discuss this stuff with the doctor. If you are embarrassed, then just have her do it. As you have probably discovered by now, after about age 18, women spend far more time talking about sex than men.

And they seem to enjoy it a lot more.

One last thing. The kind of sex referred to in this section is regular, old-timey sex. If your sex is "alternative" and involves buffet items, electronic devices, and rodeo equipment, or if you are into activities such as gymnastic sex (uneven parallel bars, pole vaults, pummel horse, ropes/rings, floor exercises, bungee cords etc.), then its probably best to cool it on these activities until after she's done expecting. Putting a hold on such activity might give you more time to figure out why you and she are such a sick couple.

Helpful Organizations

☞ BIAM KIMF Society: 1-800-GET A CLUE
(Because I Am a Man, I Know It is My Fault)
This organization helps the man understand his insensitive nature.

☞ The International Men's Association: 1-800-ADMIT IT
An association, lead and staffed by women, for the benefit of helping the man understand his faults.

☞ American College of Objective Assessment of Men: 1-800-YOUREPIGS
A valuable resource of scientific data objectively examining the role of men in today's society.

☞ The Directory of the U.S. Department of Men's Issues
1-800-WHOCARES
An entire department of the U.S. government dedicated to issues concerning medical and psychological needs of the hundreds of millions of men in the United States. (Tip: When calling, you may have to wait awhile. "Jim" is only one guy you know.)

Chapter 4: What to know about diet and lifestyle

"Look pal; you need to face reality. Life, as you know it, is over. Therefore, you better get your head on straight. Because if you don't, you'll regret it - maybe not today, maybe not tomorrow, but soon and for the rest of your life"

Bad habits

Question: *Now, that she is expecting, the doctor told her that she should quit smoking, stop alcohol, and eat a healthy diet. But I'm not the one who is pregnant. So is it O.K. if I continue to smoke, drink liquor, and eat whatever I want?*

Answer: No.

Question: *But wonder if she didn't know about it?*

Answer: She'll know.

Question: *But wonder if I was really good at hiding it?*

Answer: Look pal; you need to face reality. Life, as you know it, is over. Therefore, you better get your head on straight. Because if you don't, you'll regret it - maybe not today, maybe not tomorrow, but soon and for the rest of your life.

Question: *I know that she has to quit smoking because she's expecting. But I'm not going to stop, regardless what she, her family, the doctor, you, or anyone else says. What about that?*

Answer: Well, it's your prerogative, Mr. Cro-Magnon. You just need to be aware that you are making things much more difficult for her to stop. And because cigarette smoking by the expectant mother may be extremely harmful to her unborn child, you will have to shoulder some of the blame for any resulting problem that occurs.

If you are so weak that you can't quit smoking to improve the chances of a healthy child, then at least try to smoke outside. Respect what she's going through, and don't puff away in her face.

Geez! Have a little compassion, man!

Think about it. No one is denying the pain and hardship that you are experiencing when she's expecting. But at some point, even you have to realize that she is going through a nine-month assault on her body, with the final event of delivering a living melon through her cervix. If you still don't get it, try imagining the delivery of any kind of large fruit through your . . . well . . . maybe now you get the picture.

The point is, surely you can at least make some attempt to help her avoid cigarette smoke, and help her break the stranglehold of an addiction.

And if in the end, you both stop smoking, congratulations! You've succeeded at one of the toughest challenges around. You will have become a real man. Your next obstacle will be to stay off tobacco after the baby arrives. You might consider gum-chewing or sunflower seeds or biting your nails until your fingers bleed.

Good luck!

Question: *She is expecting, and she just drank a beer. The doctor told her not to drink alcohol. How do I punish her?*

Answer: Before you get all Neanderthal, you need the facts. First of all, it is true that most doctors will recommend that she should not drink any alcohol when she is expecting. Alcohol is a drug. And virtually all drugs should be avoided during pregnancy unless absolutely necessary.

Secondly, heavy drinking during pregnancy is a leading cause of mental retardation and birth defects. Therefore, this is a serious matter.

However, if she is a social drinker, or occasional user, she may have a tough time stopping - if for no other reason than because she is being told not to do something that she used to enjoy. (And it should be remembered, a considerable number of pregnancies involved alcohol at some point.)

If your partner does take a drink, do not freak out. A small amount of alcohol on rare occasions is not considered to be a major health problem by many health professionals. It is large and continuous amounts of substance abuse which are most often considered harmful.

Finally, remember that any "punishment" you deliver (physical or mental) will probably only breed resentment. Chances are it won't help the situation.

Therefore, a more practical approach might be to realize that her difficulty may be increased if her friends and/or family continues to drink around her. Perhaps a heart-to-heart talk with Sheila - her "sobriety-challenged" friend - might be a good place to start. Explain that for the next nine months, everyone needs to work together for the well-being of the child.

So before delivery, work with her friends. After delivery, you can go back to thinking her friends are worthless trash, and they can go back to thinking you are a lazy, inconsiderate boob.

The point is, you are her partner and the child's father. As such, you are responsible for supporting and helping her as much as possible. At the very least, if you see that your drinking is a dangerous temptation to her, then you need to stop too - or at least stop around her. Remember: the sacrifices you make are being made out of the love for your partner, your baby, and ultimately, yourself. If you use these ideas as your anchor, the entire situation should ultimately become more livable for all involved.

And then maybe you won't feel the need to drink so much.

Diet and Cravings

Question: *I've heard for so many years about the whole "Pickles and Ice Cream" food craving thing, yet she is still eating the same foods she always did. Is something wrong?*

Answer: Of course not! Not all women will experience cravings, and it is not certain when they will appear, for how long, or just how bizarre they will be.

If she does develop strange cravings, you may be asked to make a run to the market. Try not to view this as a chore. Humor her cravings. After all, how many times will you get to witness an actual human being eating a pickle, peanut butter, and mustard sandwich.

And don't expect her cravings to be consistently the same thing, either. Today's bean dip and peaches can become tomorrow's yogurt and Tabasco sauce.

Question: *I've heard that once she's expecting, she may want to eat dirt and rocks. Is this real?*

Answer: Pica is the word that refers to a depraved appetite, and can sometimes occur during pregnancy. Pica is well described in horses and is classified according to what is being consumed. For example, a desire to eat soil or sand is known as geophagia, a desire to eat wood is known as lignophagia, a desire to eat bones is known as osteophagia, a desire to eat feces is known as coprophagia, and a desire to eat a battleship with wheels is known as Buickophagia. (O.K.. We made the last one up. But the others are actual scientific terms - really!).

These bizarre cravings may have many potential causes. For example, she could just be nuts. In this case, stay away from beaches, sandboxes, and quarries.

On the other hand, it could represent hormonal changes, or an inborn response when her body detects the need for supplemental minerals to help in the rapid replication of cellular growth. Finally, at least in horses, pica sometimes represents anemia, and/or worm burdens.

So if she does develop symptoms suggestive of pica, feel free to tell everyone that you read this book, and inquire if she needs a thorough evaluation for worms.

Both she, and the obstetrician, will be appreciative of your knowledge and input.

Finally, such depraved appetites may not fit any known category. For example, one of this book's authors experienced a similar situation that every time he lit a cigar (even in another room), his expecting wife was overtaken by the desire to eat the cigar. It became the food equivalent of a loaded potato skin. This lasted only a few weeks, during which she succeeded in resisting the temptation to eat cigars. Then, it disappeared like all of the other bizarre cravings. Shortly afterward, she is now back to hating the smell of cigars, and encouraging their new baby to feel the same way.

Finally, keep in mind that some of the hormonal changes going on during the pregnancy are really screwing with her mind. And while you may think she deserves it after all those years of her screwing with yours, you need to roll with the changes and always be supportive.

And you might also hide the shovels.

Chapter 5: What to know about Month # 1

"It is important to understand that nausea and heaving during pregnancy occurs during two distinct time periods. First of all, it may occur when she eats. Secondly, it may occur when she doesn't eat."

Question: *She has been expecting for about a month. She is sleepy, fatigued, bloated, nauseated, and has heartburn and indigestion. She salivates and urinates all the time. She says she can already tell she is putting on weight. I can't tell any difference. She wants me to honestly tell her what I think about her appearance. What do I say?*

Answer: Congratulations! You are already half way there. Remember your statement that "I can't tell any difference." This will be a recurrent theme for the next nine months. At no point should you ever, under any circumstances, tell her the truth, regardless how much she morphs before you. Think of this as an ongoing game where the object is to never admit that you ever notice any difference in her appearance at any point in the pregnancy - no matter what she says, no matter what she looks like, and no matter how persuasive she is in wanting you to tell her the truth. You must remember that she does not want the truth. And you do not win points by being Mr. Honest. As far as you are concerned, she never changes.

Question: *She threw up in the sink this morning while she was brushing her teeth. What's up with that?*

Answer: It's called morning sickness, and it's not pretty - for anyone. During this phase, the slightest thing can set the whole works backwards, sending forward things back up in reverse. Some women don't need a stimulus, and just wake up and bolt for the bathroom at the break of dawn. Other women find that tooth brushing can set off a gag reflex. And when it happens, it happens quickly, buddy.

And finally, yet other pregnant women may get nauseous if they even just think about certain nasty things like eggs, or Cheez Wiz sandwiches. This may be followed by vomiting, or just dry heaves.

So what can you do?

Just be a gentleman and offer to hold her hair back for her.

Morning sickness usually sputters out around the third month. The important thing to remember is that it is only temporary. But during this time, especially if you wear nice pajamas, you may want to eat your Cheez Wiz after she goes to sleep, or perhaps in another zip code.

Question: *People have been telling me that she may be eating a lot of crackers when she's expecting. Why?*

Answer: Crackers are often recommended for soothing the expectant mother's stomach, and are most commonly recommended during the first trimester. Most women's stomachs will settle down, later in the pregnancy.

Some will not.

It's kind of like digestive roulette.

It is important to understand that nausea and heaving during pregnancy occurs during two distinct time periods. First of all, it may occur when she eats. Secondly, it may occur when she doesn't eat.

So you only need to be prepared during these times.

Hopefully, this clarifies this very important issue.

The cracker in question is usually a saltine type, since they are largely void of flavor, and expand in the stomach quickly. It might be wise to purchase a box of crackers ahead of time, for those times when the fetus decides it wants something to eat ***now***, and it's not meal time. Alternatively, you might find a local restaurant that gives away free basketfuls of individually packaged crackers. Although all businesses love to give away free food, you might consider at least ordering a small diet coke, or a bowl of tomato soup. After all, you certainly don't want to take advantage of the good will of others.

Question: *The doctor told her she needs to take prenatal vitamins to improve the health of the child. Therefore, in addition to her bee pollen, herbs, and minerals, shouldn't she take two vitamins, so that the kid will be twice as healthy?*

Answer: Hold on there, supplement breath.

First of all, in well-developed nations, a vitamin supplement is of questionable benefit in most people. So taking twice as much of something that doesn't help is basically worthless, (except to perhaps the vitamin industry):

Two x (Zero benefit + money to vitamin company) =

Zero benefit + two times as much money to vitamin company

The point is, eating a well-balanced diet that contains necessary vitamins and minerals provides the optimum chance of improved health. And most important, in the United States, the dietary and lifestyle factors that have most to do with good health is the ***avoidance*** of bad foods and bad habits, rather than the intake of good vitamins.

In other words, bee pollen doesn't solve a pack of non-filtered cigarettes, two triple cheese burgers, a large box of grease/salt soaked fries, and two six packs of cheap beer (even if they are "lite.")

Secondly, too much of certain vitamins can be toxic, particularly to the fetus. So if a pill has toxic levels of a particular vitamin, taking two will only double the toxic effects.

Thirdly, many over the counter vitamins, herbs, and minerals are often not well regulated. So you should always check with your pharmacist to be sure that the supplement you are taking is safe during pregnancy, and is manufactured by a reputable company.

Finally, having said all this, it is true that some people have medical conditions that benefit from vitamin supplementation. This appears to be so in pregnancy. Specifically, folic acid, for example, appears to substantially reduce the risks of certain types of birth defects.

So the best advice may come from your doctor. But if you and your partner are sexually active, and not using birth control, and she hasn't seen her obstetrician, then you may want to take some preliminary measures on your own. Talk to the pharmacist about starting her on a reputable prenatal multivitamin, with at least 800 mcg of folic acid (folate).

What a great gift idea!

Optimally, this should be taken months before conception. And after she is pregnant, the obstetrician may recommend another, more expensive prenatal supplement.

And you have yet another great gift idea!

Question: *I have been nauseated ever since* ***she's*** *been expecting. Could I be having morning sickness?*

Answer: Male morning sickness is sometimes referred to as "couvade" (French - "to hatch"). This condition involves psychosomatic symptoms of partners of pregnant women involving anywhere from 11% to 65% of expectant fathers.

CHAPTER 5: Month #1

The most common symptoms include changes in appetite, nausea, lack of sleep and weight gain.

However, you might also remember that many other things are likely going on at this time. These things include the following:

* A moody companion
* A nauseated, and vomiting companion
* Loss of your life as you know it
* Countless current, and future financial bills
* Closer contact with family

The point is, you may have other reasons to feel sick.

Chapter 6: What to know about Month # 2

"*But this is not a reasonable world*"

Question: *She has been expecting for about two months. She says she can definitely tell she is putting on weight. She is sleepy, fatigued, bloated, nauseated, and has heartburn and indigestion. She salivates and urinates all the time. Now, she is also breaking out with acne, and has colored stretch marks on her belly. She wants me to honestly tell her what I think about her appearance. What do I say?*

Answer: Remember the lesson of Chapter 5. At no point should you ever, under any circumstances, tell her the truth. As far as you are concerned, her looks have not changed.

Question: *Are her breasts going to get bigger?*

Answer: Yes. Breasts are a big part of the whole pregnancy situation. And as her belly grows, so do her breasts. Her nipples may change as well, becoming sensitive at times, and even leaking breast milk as the delivery of the baby draws closer.

So while she's expecting, your feelings about her breasts may change. Being asked to share something which you hold so sacred is often difficult. And you may feel slightly jilted.

If this occurs, you should try to remember the true biological purpose of those breasts. But then again, you may also remember that with regard to sharing, there ain't but one of you on this side of the womb for many months.

Enjoy!

Question: *I am worried about my wife getting stretch marks that might stay around forever, even after she's done with the whole delivery situation. Does this always happen?*

Answer: Imagine a deflated soccer ball being inserted into her belly, and then suddenly inflated. The skin is not used to being stretched that much, and this may create breakages in the skin contour - like how the outside of a melon cracks when it gets too big.

If you are concerned with the appearance of your partner's body after the baby comes, keep it to yourself. However, if you are the brave type, you can try to discuss this with her. Maybe if she knows your feelings, she can consult her doctor for ways to possibly reduce the stretching. Certain creams may help, but they are not a guarantee.

The best philosophy to have is to accept your partner, and all of the changes that her body is undergoing. Our society often places too much of an emphasis on appearance, and the pressure to look perfect is sometimes daunting. Don't damage your partner's self esteem by being unduly critical of something which is really out of her control.

Love and understand her and everything about her, and maybe she won't give you such a hard time about your nasty toe nails, love handles, nose hairs, ear hairs, etc. And if she ever does mention the loss of your scalp hair, you can always remind her about those stretch marks, and how there is no such thing as a stretch mark transplant.

After all, unless you can make her feel crummy about herself after she makes you feel crummy about yourself, what is the point of a relationship?

Question: *Once I was over the shock of finding out she was expecting, I found myself excited about the whole pregnancy situation. I wanted to show her how much I cared. So, for her birthday, I bought her jumper cables for her car. Now, suddenly, I'm the bad guy. What happened?*

Answer: First of all, the fact that she is pregnant means that you have given her a child. And that ought to be gift enough.

Secondly, don't be misled. You gave a great gift. The problem here is that she is being irrational.

Because, in the most loving, but yet practical of ways, your gift of jumper cables was among the wonderful ways to say "I care." Unfortunately, you need to understand that, apparently, women have found it necessary to catagorize gifts into "holiday gifts," and "practical gifts."

And while as a "holiday gift" can be given on any day, a

"practical gift" can never be given on a holiday.

For example, if you give a gift such as jumper cables, on a non-holiday, she (and her friends) will be very appreciative that you have demonstrated such love and concern for her safety. However, if you give the same gift on a holiday, irrespective of your sincerity, this will only encourage her, and her family and friends, to tag you with that ill-deserved "insensitive" label again.

And they will talk about it.

So the basic rule is this: yes, it is a great idea to give her gifts that help preserve her safety during the pregnancy. Jumper cables, a car phone, a security system for the house, and even a beeper are great ideas for a gift. And in any reasonable world, she would be appreciative of any gift, regardless of what it was, or when it was given. And, in a reasonable world, she would be ecstatic about your loving intent.

But this is not a reasonable world.

So put your feelings aside and don't try to be original or caring. If you do give gifts because you care about her health, safety, and life, then give them on non-holidays. On holidays, just stick to the same old tired gifts you've always had to give, such as flowers.

Because apparently, giving things that are cut for the purpose of dying in a few days is of more sentimental value than your concerns as to protecting her livelihood.

Chapter 7: What to know about Month # 3

"Your room is history."

Question: *She has been expecting for about three months. She is definitely putting on weight, and looks like her uterus is housing a plumb. She is sleepy, fatigued, bloated, nauseated, and has heartburn and indigestion. She salivates and urinates all the time. Her breasts seem larger. Now she has also broken out with total body acne, has major colored stretch marks on her belly, and has developed varicose veins. She wants me to honestly tell her what I think about her appearance. What do I say?*

Answer: Lie. Remember the lesson of Chapter 5. At no point should you ever, under any circumstances, tell her the truth. As far as you are concerned, her looks have not changed.

Question: *She is already asking me about baby names and color schemes for the nursery. And I'm the kind of person who can't decide what I want to eat for lunch. Do we really need to plan all this stuff so far in advance?*

Answer: No, but it is likely that your partner will become obsessed with the peripheral issues of the whole pregnancy situation much sooner than you will. So while you may hear her say a hundred times about how "I'm not ready to be a mother," she is certainly more than ready to remodel virtually the entire house - right now!

You should remember that many women have been planning for this time for most of their lives. And her need to prepare the nest is due an inborn instinct, imprinted on her brain cells at birth.

It is also due to the years of brainwashing by her mother, grandmothers, and vendors of baby consumer goods.

So don't be put off by her enthusiasm. If you're not the type who plans things that far in advance, suggest that she compile all of this information in a document report, with a presentation of her final proposals in a few months. And emphasize that this is not simply a way to delay the process until the NBA Finals are over. Otherwise, you may find yourself spending your time listening to the "which is more important" lecture for the next few months, instead of watching great hoops.

Question: *I just want to get it over with. What is the best way to decide the baby's name?*

Answer: Start by getting some baby name books at the bookstore. When you are deciding, please try to remember that the name you choose is something your child will have to live with for a long time. So don't get too cute. Names like Perky, Muffin, and Bambi may seem precious now, but in reality, it just makes it more difficult if your boy wants to grow up to be Senator. Also, choosing wimp names with a lot of syllables (and you know what they are) just means that your kid will probably spend the first few decades of life having his glasses, and face, broken on a daily basis.

Also, naming your child after a character such as ‘, ँ, or ˜ may have symbolic meaning. But it makes it really hard for your girl to sign checks in the future.

Wait a minute, maybe that's not such a bad . . .

Finally, be prepared for the family name battles. If you are a proud, strapping young man, you may want to establish your well-deserved immortality by naming your son after yourself.

Hey, it's your prerogative, Mr. Cro-Magnon.

Conversely, she may feel obligated to name the kid after ***her*** relatives. This may become a problem if her relatives have names that won't exactly be hip in the new millennium (and you know what they are.) Therefore, as good as her intentions are, it is not good to saddle a teenager with an outdated name that elicits phone calls from Tombstone Sam's crematorium.

So try to stick with reasonable, current names. If your kid wants to change his name to Myrtle (or Mr. Cro-Magnon) in the future, it will be his prerogative.

Question: *Before she was expecting, we remodeled the house. I personally designed my dream work room, where I now spend most of my time at home. It is unbelievable. It has all my tools, a microwave, a portable refrigerator, a monster stereo system, and a surround-sound satellite dish television network with tons of great sports channels. I also have a mega memory, EDO RAM, computer complex - complete with direct Internet access. Although she never goes in my dream room, it was always my impression that she was just as excited as I when it was finally complete.*

CHAPTER 7: Month #3

Yesterday, she mentioned that it might make a good nursery.

What did she mean by that?

Answer: Your room is history. Consider moving your stuff into the shed or garage. Or, if you are really persuasive, you might get her to let you store your stuff for the next few years on a closet shelf or storeroom, next to the brooms.

Chapter 8: What to know about Month # 4

"Her body is going to expand considerably in the coming months, as will your credit card balance."

Question: *She has been expecting for about four months. She looks like her uterus is housing an orange. She is sleepy, fatigued, bloated, and has heartburn and indigestion. She has less nausea, and less salivation and urination. However, her breasts continue to get larger. She continues to have acne, colored stretch marks on her belly, and varicose veins. Now she also has nasal congestion, nosebleeds, stuffy ears, bleeding gums and swelling of her arms and legs. She wants me to honestly tell her what I think about her appearance. What do I say?*

Answer: Continue to lie. Remember the lesson of Chapter 5. At no point should you ever, under any circumstances, tell her the truth. As far as you are concerned, her looks have not changed.

Question: *My wife seems to be spending a fortune on maternity clothes. Is this really necessary?*

Answer: Every couple in the world has their own rules about clothes shopping. Maternity wear is just an extension of the traditional fashion situation. The bottom line is; yes, she's going to need maternity clothes. Her body is going to expand considerably in the coming months, as will your credit card balance.

Maternity clothes needn't be expensive, but they certainly can be. A woman's fashion sense concerning her normal wardrobe can definitely carry over to her maternity wardrobe. Some very smart clothing designers and marketing people have certainly gotten hip to this situation, and as a result, maternity boutiques and catalogs are in abundant supply, and ready to help you unload a whole big wad of your cash. But before you take out another mortgage on the house, you might try to convince her that it is fiscally unwise to buy designer maternity clothes, since they will only be used for a few months.

You probably won't get anywhere. But she'll get a good laugh out of it.

There are alternatives, of course, including consignment shops, thrift stores, or allowing your Aunt Milly to use her sewing machine to create the most hideous garment ever designed.

Also, take a good, long look at that old table cloth you never use. A snip here, and a snip there just might save you enough money to make that car payment.

So, if you can afford it, encourage the purchase of some nice maternity outfits, which will help your partner feel more positive and, in general, sporty. But at least put up some resistance, just so you can delude yourself that you have some input into the whole pregnancy situation.

Question: *Despite my objections, she just spent a fortune on maternity clothes. But now, all she wears are my clothes. What is going on?*

Answer: First of all, your objections were well founded. It makes no sense that she just spent $100.00 on a designer outfit, only to spend her waking hours walking around in ***your*** favorite, lucky sweat shirt, and ***your*** pants - tied together with ***your*** shoe strings.

Secondly, as you have probably figured out, it is socially acceptable for her to wear men's clothes anytime. Women can do that. But let you go out just one Saturday night in her stockings and heals, and suddenly you're the strange one.

She gets compliments. You get a DSM III classification.

Question: *She's been pregnant for four months, and all she wants to do is sleep. Is this going to last during the whole pregnancy situation?*

Answer: During the second trimester of pregnancy (sometimes referred to as "The Golden Trimester") it is likely that she will feel less physically unpleasant. However, as each day goes by, she is becoming more of a walking duality. Her nutritional requirements are for two, because her metabolism is for two. Therefore, she may need the sleep of two. Don't be surprised if she turns in at nine at night, and rises at nine the next morning . . . you know . . . a lot like you sleep.

Furthermore, you may find that ***she*** may be the one to hog the couch for naps during the day. Fortunately, this is usually temporary. During the third trimester, she may feel more energetic so that you can have the couch back for your important work, such as monitoring the progress of the National Football League, or listening to those interesting callers on C-SPAN.

Question: *Yesterday, she forgot where she put her watch. Today, she pulled her car out of the driveway, but returned and asked me where she was going. Is she losing her mind?*

Answer: Increased forgetfulness can often occur during the whole pregnancy situation. But be assured that the forgetfulness is selective. For example, it is true that she may forget where she put things, or forget what she is doing. However, when it comes to remembering how you once went out with her ex-best friend seven years ago, her memory will be just fine.

Chapter 9: What to know about Month #5

"That's your job"

Question: *She has been expecting for about five months. She looks like her uterus is housing a grapefruit. She is sleepy, fatigued, bloated, and has heartburn and indigestion. She has less nausea, and less salivation and urination. However, her breasts continue to get larger. She continues to have acne, colored stretch marks on her belly, varicose veins, nasal congestion, nosebleeds, stuffy ears, bleeding gums and swelling of her arms and legs. Now she also has darkening of the skin of her face and abdomen, as well as belly pain, backache, and leg cramps. I have taken your advice, and have never admitted that I have noticed any change in her whatsoever. But, I'm starting to feel a little silly. She wants me to honestly tell her what I think about her appearance. What do I say?*

Answer: Stay the course. Continue to lie. Remember the lesson of Chapter 5. At no point should you ever, under any circumstances, tell her the truth. As far as you are concerned, her looks have not changed. Yes, you may feel silly. But your feelings are not the issue. Her feelings are the issue. Remember, if you do tell the truth, you will hurt her feelings, and it is you who will feel the pain.

Question: *We were planning a business trip. What about traveling on a plane?*

Answer: With regard to plane trips, the main thing to consider is her comfort. In other words, will the seat size and leg room be sufficient, or will she and the baby be wedged in like frat boys in a phone booth?

CHAPTER 9: Month #5

So you might consider reserving an exit row seat. And if your little puffball has added a few extra pounds too many during the pregnancy, you might try:

(1) reserving the entire exit row.

Remember also that her bladder may be in overdrive. And plane flights don't always accommodate one's immediate need to visit the bathroom.

So, you may want to:

(1) reserve the entire exit row,

(2) next to the nearest bathroom.

Finally, if you and she are the kind of people who hate to fly, and feel all freaky, panicky and paranoid, even when she is not expecting, then you may want to postpone your flying plans until after the baby comes.

Otherwise, you may want to:

(1) reserve the entire exit row,

(2) next to the nearest bathroom,

(3) next to the friendly flight attendant with the friendly wrist restraints.

Question: *We were planning a trip to see her parents. What about a long trip in a car?*

Answer: Most women are safe to travel in planes or cars until near the end of their pregnancy, unless instructed otherwise by the doctor. During the last few months, it is probably not wise to take trips far from home. Otherwise, the unexpected may happen. And you may find it "uncomfortable" that the only one around to help deliver the child on Route 666, at 12:00 Midnight, is Hadie, the toothless former nurse's aid, who hasn't had human contact since the Salem witch trials.

From a comfort standpoint, long trips in the car present a lot of the same difficulties as flying, except that you can always pull the car over and stop - a practice which most airlines tend to frown upon. Cars can be made a little more comfortable, depending on how many people are traveling. You may even suggest that she drive; she'd be guaranteed to have more legroom that way. It is not, however, recommended that the expectant mother drive late at night, particularly if you are unclear where you are going. Because it might be dangerous to be driving in the dark through uncertain lands, while steadfastly refusing to use a road map.

That's your job.

It is also a good idea to keep plenty of snacks in the car, especially crackers if you're traveling during the first trimester. If your partner is experiencing cravings, simply stop at a convenience store, purchase one of every item that they have, and hope for the best. If you are planning a trip during the first trimester and your partner is experiencing nausea and vomiting, suggest a nice quiet weekend at home.

You'll thank yourself for it later.

Question: *I have heard about people putting headphones on the mother's belly so that the baby can hear music inside the womb. Does this really work?*

Answer: It is a known fact that babies in the womb can hear as early as the end of the second trimester. What they actually decipher is impossible to determine, because they generally don't talk about it. But it is a universal belief that all beautiful creatures love beautiful music.

"Beautiful" is, of course, an individual preference. If you think "Metallica" and "MegaDeth" are beautiful, then by all means, go for it. But if you do, first remember to keep the volume reasonable. Secondly, don't be surprised if your child bangs its head a lot after birth.

Country music has advantages in that it typically has a good solid, easily defined beat that junior can get into. You may find that your unborn child kicks in synchrony with the music, giving you the warm secure knowledge that your child is first learning to line dance/clog on the floor of a uterus.

Alternatively, many couples choose soothing classical music or jazz for their baby's listening pleasure. Bebop may be O.K. too.

However, after birth, when your baby first begins to make gibberish noises, it may be difficult to determine if she is just making baby talk, or if she just beeped, when she should have bopped.

But if your child continues to utter meaningless gibberish, even as it grows older, it may be well on the way to a successful jazz singing career, or a seat in the House of Representatives.

Chapter 10: What to know about Month #6

"The best thing about pregnancy is that it only occurs in women."

Question: *She has been expecting for about six months. She looks like her uterus is housing a coconut. She is sleepy, fatigued, bloated, and has heartburn and indigestion. She has less nausea, and less salivation and urination. However, her breasts continue to get larger. She continues to have acne, colored stretch marks on her belly, varicose veins, nasal congestion, nosebleeds, stuffy ears, bleeding gums, swelling of her arms and legs, darkening of the skin of her face and abdomen, belly pain, backache, and leg cramps. Now she says her belly "itches." I have taken your advice, and have never admitted that I have noticed any change in her whatsoever. But, this is ridiculous. I have got to acknowledge something. She wants me to honestly tell her what I think about her appearance. What do I say?*

Answer: As difficult as it may be, you must continue to lie. Remember the lesson of Chapter 5. At no point should you ever, under any circumstances, tell her the truth. As far as you are concerned, her looks have not changed. You only have a few months to go. If you find yourself growing weak, and want to give some type of response, try to use the word "glow" a lot - as in "Geez honey, the only difference I can tell is that you seem to have an almost angelic glow." Although she may want to, it will be difficult for her to cuss you out, in person (especially after you had just sited a biblical reference).

Question: *This is our first child. All of us (including me, our doctor, and her family) have tried to assure her that everything* *will be O.K. However, her coworkers find it necessary to scare her to death on a daily basis. They tell story after story of horrible experiences during pregnancy. Furthermore, they have convinced her that our baby will never eat, never sleep, and will likely be born possessed. Why do her (supposed) friends act this way?*

Answer: Although a closely guarded secret, new mothers must go through a hazing ritual. Any woman who is considering entering into the club of motherhood must endure nine months of horror stories by her friends, usually followed by a "reassuring" statement such as:

> *"But this probably won't happen to you."*

And you can't do much about it, because these stories come from her trusted family and friends. And since you are a man, how can you possibly understand what she is going through?

Gestational Diabetes Mellitus
(diabetes that only occurs during pregnancy)

Question: *She has been expecting for about 26 weeks. Yesterday, she took a test where she drank some syrupy stuff to* *see if she had diabetes mellitus. She apparently failed. Now she has to go back and drink more "glucose," and have more blood drawn. She has never had diabetes before, and no one in her family has had diabetes. What is glucose anyway? Why does she have to drink that stuff? Isn't this a big bunch of trouble, and a big waste of time and money?*

Answer: Glucose is the kind of sugar that is found in the blood. That is why glucose is called "blood sugar." Sucrose is found in a shaker on the table. That is why sucrose is called "table sugar." Glucose is not the same as table sugar, even if blood is spilled on the table.

The first test she had was just a screening test in which she drank 50 grams of a nasty glucose solution, followed by a sugar blood level drawn after one hour. If this one hour blood sugar level is greater than 140 mg/dl, then a more complete glucose tolerance test (GTT) is often recommended. The GTT includes at least an eight hour fast, followed by a fasting blood sugar the next morning. Afterwards, she gets to drink 100 grams of the nasty glucose solution.

Glucose blood levels are then obtained 1, 2, and 3 hours later.

Yes, this is a lot of blood sticks - thus verifying the one underlying theme during the whole pregnancy situation:

> *The best thing about pregnancy is that it only occurs in women.*

CHAPTER 10: Month #6

Question: *She has been diagnosed with gestational diabetes mellitus. What caused it? Did she eat too much sugar?*

Answer: The risk factors for gestational diabetes include:

* Higher maternal age during pregnancy
* Being overweight or obese
* Family history of diabetes mellitus
* Ethnicity (Hispanics and African-Americans are at increased risk for type II or adult onset diabetes mellitus and may be at increased risk for gestational diabetes mellitus)
* Previous gestational diabetes
* Previous large child at birth (previous delivery of a baby weighing more than 9 pounds)

Although gestational diabetes mellitus may occur, even without these risk factors, glucose tolerance testing is most often recommended for at risk women from 24 to 28 weeks gestation.

Gestational diabetes mellitus is one of the most common nutritional problems that develops during pregnancy. And while eating too much sugar can sometimes increase blood sugar, eating too much sugar did not cause the underlying problem (unless it contributed to excessive weight gain during the pregnancy). This condition probably has many causes. But the main problem is that she has developed a resistance to her own insulin.

Her body is being stubborn. (What a surprise.)

And since insulin is required to lower blood sugars, this resistance to insulin's effect has caused the blood sugars to be high, particularly after meals.

Question: *She has been diagnosed with gestational diabetes. The doctor said that if it is not controlled, we may have a big kid. But I want a big kid. Can we let her blood sugars go high, so we can have a bigger kid?*

Answer: Allowing the blood sugars of the woman with gestational diabetes to be uncontrolled during pregnancy may cause the mother to have increased thirst, urination, and fetal amniotic fluid, as well as an increased rate of urinary tract infections, yeast infections, spontaneous abortions, hypertension and toxemia. If the baby does get to be too big, the mother may experience a difficult delivery, prolonged labor, vaginal wall trauma, and/or a need for a cesarian section. And the newborn may experience birth trauma such as brachial plexus injury, facial nerve injury, and cephalohematoma, as well as metabolic problems such as respiratory distress, low blood sugar, electrolyte imbalances, and an increased risk of obesity, and diabetes mellitus later in the newborn's life.

So yes, allowing the blood sugars to go uncontrolled may result in a large, fat baby at birth, and may also result in numerous complications to the mother and newborn.

And it should be remembered that a large baby does not mean that the child will grow to be a bigger, more muscular adult. In fact, evidence suggests the opposite. Babies that are born too big to women with gestational diabetes mellitus may grow up with an increased risk of obesity, and development of disease states such as diabetes mellitus.

So for those of you who would consider risking her health in the hopes of creating an NFL caliber son, with a multimillion dollar professional football contract to fund your sorry butt when you grow older, this is the wrong way to do it. Instead, your plan to encourage her to stay off her diet may cause unneeded medical complications, and will probably result in a flabby offspring, just as lazy as you.

Hey, but it's your prerogative, Mr. Cro-Magnon.

Question: *She has been diagnosed with gestational diabetes. What is the best way for blood sugars to be monitored?*

Answer: Once the diagnosis of gestational diabetes mellitus is made, one strategy is to monitor blood sugars fasting, and two hours after each meal (four times a day).

Yes, this is a lot of blood sticks. But remember:

> *The best thing about pregnancy is that it only occurs in women.*

With current technology blood sugar testing can easily be done with home glucose monitors readily found at drugstores, or even department stores. The goal is to maintain fasting blood sugars less than 90 mg/dL, and two hour after meal blood sugars less than 120 mg/dl.

Urinary ketone determination may also be recommended to determine periods of relative "starvation." During pregnancy, she has the metabolism of two, and must maintain enough calories to sustain two. And partially because women with gestational diabetes mellitus treated with diet may try a little too hard to avoid the need for insulin, a measurement of starvation states is needed.

If inadequate caloric intake occurs, and the supplies of consumed and/or stored carbohydrates are depleted, then the body has to look elsewhere for calories. Hence, the mother's fat then becomes a major source of calories. And as you may recall from your biochemistry, the breakdown of fat results in the formation of "ketones."

Because the kidneys are very efficient in clearing ketones, even if urinary ketones are moderate, it is unlikely that ketone levels in the blood are significantly elevated. However, if urinary ketones become highly positive, this may mean that the blood may become more acid-like. Therefore, maintaining urinary ketones less than moderate is a reasonable treatment goal. Such urine testing is usually recommended fasting, whenever meals are omitted, during periods of nausea or vomiting, or with medical stresses, such as during infections.

CHAPTER 10: Month #6

Another test is the total glycated hemoglobin (TGH), or hemoglobin A1C (Hgb A1C), which can be obtained on a single blood draw while at the doctor's office. These tests determine the overall blood sugar control for the previous 6 - 8 weeks. So if these tests suggest that she has had significantly high blood sugars in the past couple of months, and this is not reflective on her own blood sugar monitoring charts because she is just making up numbers instead of actually checking her blood sugars, the doctor will know.

The doctor will know.

She can run, but she cannot hide.

Question: *She has been diagnosed with gestational diabetes mellitus. The doctor said it is important that she avoid sugars such as fruit juices, pizza, and raw carrots, but that table sugar might be O.K.*

What is the doctor talking about?

Answer: In general, women with gestational diabetes mellitus should be encouraged to adhere to healthy, low concentrated sweet diets. If high blood pressure and/or swelling occurs, then reduction in dietary sodium may also be important.

However, some unique recommendations include a greater percentage of fat in the diet to reduce the after meal blood sugar effects of carbohydrates. Furthermore, it is important to understand that different foods have different effects on blood sugar. The blood sugar response to mixed meals is most dependent on the type, and amount (or percentage) of carbohydrates. The glycemic response to isolated foods may be anticipated by the "glycemic index."

The Glycemic Index is the amount of rise in blood sugar, after ingestion of a fixed amount of a certain food. For example, if 100 grams of glucose ingestion caused a rise in blood sugar by 50 mg/dl, then this is the standard by which other foods are compared. If ingestion of another food only caused a 25 mg/dl rise in blood sugar, then the GI for this food would be 50%. (Please note that sucrose - table sugar - has a GI of about 50%.)

As can be seen from the chart, the effect of certain foods on blood sugar is not necessarily obvious.

For example, most people would have guessed that foods such as sugared soft drinks would jack up blood sugars. However, fewer know that fruit juices can as well.

Just because it is a "natural" sugar does not make it any less a sugar.

Furthermore, few people would have guessed that cornflakes, raw carrots, and potatoes would raise blood sugar more than ice cream. That is because ice cream is largely fat. And fat is not sugar. On the other hand, the other foods mentioned are composed of carbohydrates that are easily, and quickly broken down in the gut, with significant effects on blood sugar.

CHAPTER 10: Month #6

GLYCEMIC INDEX OF SOME FOODS

100%: Glucose

80 - 90%: Cornflakes, carrots, potatoes (instant or mashed), honey

70 - 79%: Whole wheat or whole meal bread, white rice, potatoes

60 - 69%: White bread, shredded wheat, brown rice, raisins, beets, bananas, mars bar

50 - 59%: Bran, many biscuits, white spaghetti, sweet corn, green peas, potato chips, sucrose, pastry

40 - 49%: Oat meal, whole meal spaghetti, sweet potatoes, navy beans, dry peas, grapes, oranges

30 - 39%: Butter beans, chick and black eye peas, ice cream, milk, yogurt, tomatoes, apples, pears

20 - 29%: Sausage, kidney beans, lentils, fructose, peaches, grapefruit, plums, cherries

10 - 19%: Soybeans, peanuts

And if that were not confusing enough, studies have shown (and practical experience has confirmed) that one of the foods that increase blood sugars the most is pizza.

Doesn't pizza have a lot of fat?

Therefore, from a practical standpoint, perhaps the best method to determine the glycemic properties of food is through intensive home glucose monitoring. Monitoring blood sugars four times a day, seven days a week, will quickly educate women with gestational diabetes mellitus as to which foods result in after meal high blood sugar.

And if a certain food particularly increases blood sugar, then she shouldn't eat that anymore.

("Doctor, doctor, every time I hit my head, I get a headache. What should I do?" " Don't hit your head anymore," replied the doctor.)

If she feels that she just ***has*** to eat foods with high glycemic index, she could try to incorporate them into mixed meals. This may blunt blood sugar excursions. For example, eating potatoes or bread alone may cause unacceptable elevations in blood sugar, sometimes reaching the point where she may have to start insulin injections. However, if high glycemic index foods are eaten, mixed with high fat foods such as steak and butter, then insulin treatment may not be necessary.

Another way to limit after meal high blood sugars (and limit urinary ketosis) is to spread the daily caloric consumption to six small meals a day.

But the optimal way to possibly avoid the whole gestational diabetes situation is to be sure that she is at ideal body weight, before she gets pregnant.

But that is a war is between you and her.

Question: *She has been diagnosed with gestational diabetes. Shouldn't she be on a big-time weight reduction diet?*

Answer: Pregnancy is not the time to enter into a weight reduction program. All mothers with gestational diabetes mellitus should eat healthy and regular meals. But while as many women typically gain about 25 pounds over the course of pregnancy, some overweight pregnant mothers may not gain any more weight during pregnancy, and may actually lose weight while on a gestational diabetes mellitus diet. This is usually acceptable, as long as the weight loss is not excessive, is not due to an underlying illness, is not due to uncontrolled blood sugars, and as is not associated with positive urinary ketones.

And it is important to note that many overweight women find that if they adhere to an appropriate diet ***during*** pregnancy, they may eventually weigh less ***after*** the pregnancy, than before the pregnancy.

Good for her. Good for you.

Question: *Should blood sugars be checked after delivery?*

Answer: Most mothers with gestational diabetes mellitus will not need to monitor blood sugars after delivery. However, this should be left up to the doctors.

As good as this book is, doctors should still be involved.

Question: *If she has gestational diabetes during pregnancy, will she have diabetes mellitus after delivery?*

Answer: In the vast majority of cases, if she did not have diabetes mellitus before pregnancy, it is unlikely she will have diabetes after delivery. However, about 35-50% of women with history of gestational diabetes mellitus will develop type II, or adult onset diabetes at some point in their lifetime. The best way to avoid diabetes mellitus after delivery, is for her to strive to obtain ideal body weight and enter into a regular physical exercise program.

The bottom-line is that if she wants to maximize her chances of avoiding the gestational diabetes mellitus next time, then she will need to adhere to favorable lifestyle habits long after delivery. Otherwise, she will, almost undoubtedly, develop gestational diabetes mellitus with future pregnancies.

And even if she does all the right things, and makes all the sacrifices and effort, she still may have to go through the whole diet and blood sugar monitoring thing again during future pregnancies - thus again confirming:

> *The best thing about pregnancy is that it only occurs in women.*

Chapter 11: What to know about Month # 7

"After all, why waste your time? She's the one who's expecting"

Question: *She has been expecting for about seven months. She looks like her uterus is housing a cantaloupe. She is sleepy, fatigued, bloated, and has heartburn and indigestion. She has less nausea, and less salivation and urination. However, her breasts continue to get larger. She continues to have acne, colored stretch marks on her belly, varicose veins, nasal congestion, nosebleeds, stuffy ears, bleeding gums, swelling of her arms and legs, darkening of the skin of her face and abdomen, belly pain, backache, and leg cramps. Her belly "itches." Now she complains of clumsiness, loss of balance, false labor pains, and leaky breasts. I have really tried to take your advice, and have never admitted that I have noticed any change in her whatsoever. But my resistance is fading. I find myself desperately wanting to tell the truth. She wants me to honestly tell her what I think about her appearance. What do I say?*

Answer: Now is the time to read, and reread the lessons of Chapter 5. You are just weeks away from victory. All you have to do is to avoid, under any circumstances, telling her the truth. As far as you are concerned, her looks have not changed. You only have a few months to go.

Question: *Every time she tells me that the baby is kicking, she insists that I put my hand on her belly. But when I tell her I don't really feel anything, I feel like it's my fault, and that somehow, I am not adequately participating in the whole pregnancy situation. What is the problem?*

Answer: First of all, she will always be more sensitive to the baby's movements that you, because she's the one who's expecting. Therefore, it is no surprise that she is feeling the kicks more than you. Think of it this way, if the fetus was growing in your testicles, and suddenly kicked, it is likely you would feel it more than her.

Secondly, your unborn child may only kick on an intermittent basis. And this shouldn't be surprising. For example, if you were sitting in a uterine lounge chair, and were being supplied with food and drink without having to lift a finger, how much kicking would you do?

So don't be discouraged.

Also, while it may be difficult at first to feel the baby's movements in the beginning, it may become a daily occurrence after a few weeks/months. In fact, you may eventually even see the baby actually ruffling and rolling the skin of her abdomen.

That is definitely weird.

The movie "Aliens" may come to mind.

In time, the baby movement thing will become old hat to you and your partner. Other people, however, may want to feel the baby move. And while she may not always mind some stranger putting a quick hand on her belly, you might want to make sure it's okay with her before you offer to let someone "touch the merchandise."

Question: *Every time she tells me that the baby is kicking, she insists that I put my hand on her belly. But I don't really care. How do I convey this message without giving the impression that I am not enthusiastically participating in the whole pregnancy situation?*

Answer: How have you handled other situations you were suppose to care about in the past? How have you handled birthdays, anniversaries, weddings, and her family reunions (as well as your own family reunions for that matter).

If you think about it, the whole baby-kicking situation isn't that much different.

Fake it.

Question: *She is upset. We do not know the gender of our child. But her friends insist they do. On the one hand, Gertrude, an old wife, has told her we are definitely having a girl. The scientific proof is overwhelming, and based upon the fact that my partner has been carrying the baby high, and closer to the hips rather than low and out front, has noted no increase hair growth to the legs, has been sleeping with the pillow to the south, has a baby heart rate greater than 140 beats/minute, has noted no colder feet, has refused to eat the heal of a loaf of bread, has a grandmother with hair that is not gray, has had severe morning sickness early in the pregnancy, has had dramatic breast enlargement, has not been looking particularly good* *during pregnancy, has noted that a thread with a needle held over the belly moves side to side rather than in a circle, has had urine that is dull yellow rather than bright yellow and finally, it is definitely a girl because I (as the father) have not put on as much weight as my partner during the whole pregnancy situation.*

On the other hand, her friend Annie, a teacher, says that we are definitely having a boy because my partner's age at the time of conception, added to the number of the month that conception took place, is an even number. This means we are having a boy. And to confirm her case, Annie ran the numbers on the Chinese Gender Chart, and sure enough, we are definitely having a boy.

Finally, each of her other friends has their own opinion, based upon the scientific fact that "they can just tell."

And the odd thing is that every one of her friends indicates that they have never been wrong.

Whom do we believe?

Answer: Your partner is not going to want to hear this. But the only reasonable way to make any valid guess as to the gender of the child is by ultrasound, chorionic villus sampling, or amniocentesis. However, all her friends will insist that they know, without such scientific techniques. But in reality, they have no more of a chance in picking the correct gender than a flip of a coin. Having said this, as soon as it is known what the actual gender is, all those that guessed correctly will be reaffirmed as legitimate soothsayers. And all of those that guessed wrong will say something like:

> *"Well, I guessed it was a girl, but I kind of thought it was a boy."*

In other words, even if every single one of her friends were wrong, it is unlikely that they would simply come out and admit that their foolproof indicators were nothing more than speculation.

And even more surprising will be your partner. Because if ninety-nine of her friends guessed wrong, and one friend guessed right, she will not focus on how the ninety-nine were dead wrong. Instead, she will focus on how her one friend was right.

You should be so lucky.

Work Issues

Question: *How long should she continue to work?*

Answer: This will most likely be determined by her doctor, based upon her physical condition. If her blood pressure is deemed too high, or if other health issues arise, then her doctor may recommend that she cut back or stop working all together.

CHAPTER 11: Month # 7

If she is required to stay off work, it could be weeks until the baby is born. And she may get bored and restless during this time. Just imagine how restless you'd be - bed ridden for weeks on end. Then imagine being bed ridden, feeling crappy, ***and*** knowing that this huge bundle of uncertainty is about to explode from between your legs.

Makes for an attractive visual, doesn't it?

So she will definitely need your help throughout this difficult stage in the pregnancy. Make sure that she has someone around in case she needs immediate assistance. This may require flexibility in your work schedule, or may require potential work sacrifice on your part. Yes, in a perfect world, it would be best if her labor did not disrupt your work schedule. Yes, in a perfect world, when she went into labor, it would be nice if she just drove herself to the hospital, and notified you when the whole delivery situation was over.

But we do not live in a perfect world.

And to allow her to do this all on her own, without a plan to assist her, will only encourage her, and her family and friends, to tag you with that ill-deserved "insensitive" label again.

So be prepared.

Also, you may want to help her plan activities which will fend off boredom. Rent her some movies. Help her start a jigsaw puzzle. Buy her another baby name book. But most of all, try to hide all the baby mail-order catalogues, and conveniently "lose" her credit cards. Because if she has time and access, it will be difficult for her to avoid the purchase of more baby stuff. And if she does, you're stuck. Think about it. If while lying at home like a sick beached whale, she decides to order a $50 Mickey Mouse foot blanket, what are you going to do? Yelling at her at this stage will do little more than to encourage her, and her family and friends, to tag you with that ill-deserved "insensitive" label again.

Question: *She seems to be very tired and uncomfortable. She went to the doctor who said that it was medically O.K. for her to work. But she is asking if I think she should take some time off anyway. But we really need the money.*

What do I do?

Answer: Obviously if she had a medical problem that the doctor felt required her to stop working, she should stop working. However, if you really need the money, then you need to come up with a strategy that keeps her at work, without implying that you simply want to maintain the cash flow. Otherwise, you might have to justify spending money on such important things as those new bowling shoes, that latest computer software, and/or the new wheels for your car.

You may even have to explain the absurd notion as to why you haven't even considered selling the boat.

Therefore, the best approach is to use the pressures of today's expectations of women to your advantage. Play on her fears. For example, when she begins to talk about taking time off from work, simply agree that this may be a good idea. But then immediately follow-up with mentioning all the other career women you know who worked until the day of delivery. If possible, specifically, talk about a single-minded, aggressive, corporate woman that she is particularly envious of, or intimidated by. This will trigger the jealousy gene that will likely force her to continue working until the baby literally drops from the womb.

This may seem a little cruel to use this kind of psychology. But hey, at least you will be able to afford a few more bowling days out of it.

Prenatal Classes

Question: *My wife asked me to go to a "Fathers Only" class. Won't this just be a stupid waste of time?*

Answer: Yes.

That's what most real men would say if they were asked that question. Having a bunch of big hairy guys in a room talking about their new-found feelings of insecurity of fatherhood is about as entertaining as having a wisdom tooth extracted.

But if you do go, you may find that the "Fathers Only" thing is not so bad.

Such a gathering gives you a chance to consider what your new role is going to be, and how you or some stranger feels about it. And it also gives you a chance to be totally embarrassed as you express how little you know about the whole pregnancy situation, while at the same time, laughing at the other poor slobs who say some really idiotic things.

If you are lucky, you probably won't be forced to talk in front of the whole room, and you won't have to stand up and say your name like an A.A. meeting. However, you probably will be asked to use your brain (and maybe your heart) for about thirty or forty minutes. And you probably will leave feeling a lot better about everything than you did when you came in.

At least you will know that you are not an anomaly to your gender.

Question: *The hospital is offering a series of pregnancy classes. Do I need to attend all of these?*

Answer: That's all a matter of how informed you want to be about this whole pregnancy situation. A wise man once said that a little knowledge is a dangerous thing, so going to the class that appeals to you most, and ignoring all the rest, could prove hazardous.

Beware!

But, in most cases, these classes usually offer something which will benefit fathers further on up the road. For example, while you may not think you need to know anything about breast feeding, if you attend the class, you might benefit from learning some interesting facts that you probably wouldn't have otherwise known.

And you shouldn't feel guilty that you didn't already know some of this woman's stuff. After all, unless she took a class on male rectal exams, how much would she know about prostate health?

Preparation

Question: *She is seven-months pregnant, and is already getting stuff together for a "Hospital Bag." Is this really necessary? Isn't packing all this stuff ridiculous?*

Answer: Yes, a "Hospital Bag" is necessary, and it is ridiculous.

So let her pack it, rack it, stack it, and otherwise have it ready for action. Memorize the contents of the bag and what each item's purpose will be. That way, when she is in labor, and starts screaming:

"Get me the tennis balls!"

You won't stare at her in absolute befuddlement.

That won't do anyone any good.

And regardless of how useless, don't question why she needs some of the things she packed. Instead, you may want to focus on what ***you*** need. Some items you might consider include the following:

(1) Comfortable clothes. You don't want to be wearing a business suit, scuba gear, or chaps hour after hour while sitting on hideous hospital furniture while you await junior to make his big debut. So pack some of your favorite "kick around" clothes. Consequently, if you get "the call" while you're at work, you won't have trouble changing into comfy duds - 'cause' they're in the bag.

(2) Snack items. You should be prepared for the possibility that you could be trapped in a birthing suite for twenty hours or more, unable to leave her side. So since she may not be allowed to eat, it is your responsibility to bring enough food to keep you well-nourished for the both of you.

And imagine the courageousness you will display when,

despite her inability to eat while she is undergoing hour after hour of painful labor, you bravely maintain your strength by eating in front of her.

And bringing well-chosen snacks keeps you from having to rely on those dried up burgers at the hospital coffee shop. And while the hospital food machines may have snacks, how long can you afford to eat $1.00 bags of four year old peanut butter and Styrofoam crunch bars.

(3) Reading material and other forms of entertainment. Although labor and delivery may sound exciting, you might be surprised how much down time there is during the whole delivery situation.

And definitely bring the “sports on the air” section of the newspaper. Many hospital rooms have televisions. And if you plan things just right, maybe you can watch the big games while she’s in labor, and she can deliver after they’re over.

After all, why waste your time?

She’s the one who’s expecting.

Chapter 12: What to know about Month #8

"And while as you may feel that this drivel makes you out to be some kind of weenie, remember . . . well . . . come to think of it . . . you will be a weenie."

Question: *She has been expecting for about eight months. She looks like her uterus is housing a watermelon. She is sleepy, fatigued, bloated, and has heartburn and indigestion. She has less nausea, and less salivation and urination. However, her breasts continue to get larger. She continues to have acne, colored stretch marks on her belly, varicose veins, nasal congestion, nosebleeds, stuffy ears, bleeding gums, swelling of her arms and legs, darkening of the skin of her face and abdomen, belly pain, backache, and leg cramps. Her belly "itches." She complains of clumsiness, loss of balance, false labor pains, and leaky breasts. Now she is short of breath, and has a really fast heart rate. She also has hemorrhoids and her navel is about ready to explode. I have really tried to take your advice, and have never admitted that I have noticed any change in her whatsoever. But my resistance is fading. I can't take it anymore. I have got to tell her the truth. She wants me to honestly tell her what I think about her appearance. What do I say?*

Answer: You are almost there. Don't blow it. If you have had the discipline in following the advice of Chapter 5 until now, you are so far ahead of the game, that it is hard to describe. You are venturing into realms of reality few have ever experienced. Take a few breaths, say a few prayers for forgiveness, and avoid, under any circumstances, telling her the truth. As far as you are concerned, her looks have not changed. You only have one month to go.

CHAPTER 12: Month # 8

Baby Showers

Question: *My wife's friends have planned a baby shower. Do I have to go?*

Answer: There's a fifty-fifty chance that you will. If it's a "couples shower," then you'll definitely have to go. The up side is that there may be a whole bunch of other men there suffering right along with you.

Why do women insist that men suffer through baby showers, or for that matter, wedding showers, or any other kind of showers?

The answer is simple. Women need to share the rain. They want you to share experiences with them. As such, your level of caring is defined by how willing you are to endure experiences out of your element.

And the more painful the experience, the greater your demonstration of caring.

For example, baby showers are quite painful experiences. So, if you decline to attend an invitation to a couples baby shower, and if at least one other poor man slob attends, then this will encourage her, and her family and friends, to tag you with that ill-deserved "insensitive" label again. If you do attend, then you will have proven your worth as her companion - but only if you don't cause a scene. And remember, "a scene" doesn't necessarily mean throwing a fit. It can equally be a problem if you just don't pay attention, or don't get "involved."

The point is, don't plan on watching the Green Bay/Chicago game during the baby shower.

The process of the baby shower involves the opening and passing around of gifts that, often, are both completely alien and downright frightening to men. Sure, we'll understand their purpose later, after she has explained them to us. But at that moment, while in front of all of those shower guests, you will come face-to-face with the unknown world surrounding the whole baby-stuff situation. And to not know what a "onesie" or a "diaper genie" is can be an exercise in utter humiliation. (See "What words to know" in the back of the book.)

Finally, the decision as to whether it will be a "couples shower" or a "girls only" shower will probably be made by her, or her friends. The basic point is, although you may be expected to attend, you won't have much input into the whole baby shower situation.

Surprise, surprise.

Question: *My women coworkers gave me a baby shower. I have no idea what this was. Since my wife likes to open presents, I simply planned on taking the boxes home to her, without opening them. Suddenly I was the ungrateful, insensitive, bad guy. But I thought I was being sensitive. Where did I go wrong this time?*

Answer: First of all, you are a man. Therefore, by definition, you cannot be sensitive, particularly when she is expecting. Secondly, you clearly are in need of baby-shower practice. In the past, baby showers were only for women. But now, some women in the workplace will have baby showers - just for men. You need to understand that the baby shower is an opportunity for others to give gifts. It is your obligation to unwrap, and unbox all gifts. You must then discuss how, and how much you are going to use whatever you were given. The following template may be useful:

> *"Oh, this is great. We were really wanting a _____. This will be great when we are _____, and the baby is ______. That was so sweet."*

And while as you may feel that this drivel makes you out to be some kind of weenie, remember . . . well . . . come to think of it . . . you will be a weenie.

Question: *She just got back from her baby shower. I didn't have to go. However, I am curious, what are "baby shower games?" What is their purpose?*

Answer: Baby showers include sometimes bizarre, and at times, almost frightening "games" that have been practiced for decades. And surprisingly, they continue to be practiced today. Some of the more common includes the following:

(1) Mustard paper lottery: In this peculiar game, paper towels are carefully separated into square sheets, precisely along their respective serrated edges. In the center of one single sheet is placed an exact amount of mustard, and all sheets are subsequently folded. As each member of the baby shower caldron enters, they are handed a folded, separated sheet. At the end of the ritual, the sole owner of the mustard sheet is discovered, and is anointed the winner.

Of what, we do not know.

(2) Toilet paper enshroudment: In yet another paper "game" (the recurrent symbolic meaning of the paper remains unclear), a roll of toilet paper is issued to a member, who is required to savagely tear off a portion of the roll to the exact, anticipated length that would wrap around the abdominal girth of the expecting mother. The roll is then passed down to the next member, and to each subsequent member of the baby shower caldron. After all challenges have been accepted and completed, each member proceeds to wrap their portion of paper around the pregnant woman. Who so best guessed the circumference of the mother's belly wins.

Of what, we do not ask.

(3) Clothes pen chastity: This is perhaps the most medieval of games still practiced today. In this "game," each baby shower member receives a clothes' pen. Any member who discovers that another member has crossed her legs, becomes the rightful owner of that members pen. The member with the most pens wins.

Of what, we do not even venture to guess. However, if the member who is least is apt to cross her legs wins, we can only surmise that she is the one most likely to be the subject of the next baby shower.

So, what is the point of these strange on goings?

What is the ultimate purpose of these mysterious "games?"

Unfortunately, it has not as yet been revealed to the male gender. But from all the evidence from our research into these twisted practices, it can be safely be said that we don't need to know.

We don't want to know.

Be afraid!

Contractions

Question: *She is only eight-months pregnant, but complaining a lot about a clenching sensation in her crotch. Could she be in labor this soon?*

Answer: It is probable that she is having Braxton Hicks contractions. These are contractions that occur before actual labor, and usually after twenty weeks of pregnancy. They represent a flexing of the uterine muscles that can anywhere from

30 seconds to two minutes. As time goes on, these contractions may become more painful. Sometimes they may be so painful that they feel less like false labor (Braxton Hicks contractions), and more like a lawn mower in the uterus (Briggs and Stratton contractions) and/or a hand drill in the uterus (Black and Decker contractions.)

Question: *How do I know when she's having real labor?*

Answer: This is often difficult to determine. But here are some clues:

(1) If her contractions become more and more regular, and more and more painful, and she is telling you more and more she needs to go to the hospital, then she probably is having real labor.

(2) If her water bursts all over the carpet, then she probably is having real labor.

(3) If her cervix is dilated to the diameter of a man hole cover, then she probably is having real labor.

Ultrasound

Question: *I keep hearing about an ultrasound. Why haven't we had one yet?*

Answer: An ultrasound is a non-invasive procedure that may be used to determine the progression of pregnancy, and involves bouncing sound waves off the fetus to create a picture. An ultrasound may or may not be needed during the pregnancy, depending upon her clinical status, depending upon her doctor, and most of all, depending her insurance company.

Don't worry. These sound waves don't hurt the fetus. And don't feel too bad that this might wake up the little angel. Soon enough, you will discover how little it cares about bombarding you, night after sleepless night, with an entire repertoire of annoying sounds.

And remember, if it goes well, you may get a picture. They may even give you a video tape. But realize that no matter how many times you watch it, it will likely still have no interpretable sound, no plot, and no identifiable characters.

You know . . . kind of like a Fox Network sitcom.

If she does get an ultrasound, it is likely that the most you will be able to see is a tiny pulsating orb - which they will tell you is your baby.

Whether or not you choose to believe this is up to you.

Also, be prepared that early in pregnancy, since the little zygote is so deeply positioned inside its mother's body, the ultrasound technician may need to use a wand, inserted vaginally, to perform an internal ultrasound.

Which brings to mind an important lesson learned in Chapter 10:

> *"The best thing about pregnancy is that it only occurs in women."*

If a repeat is needed later in the pregnancy, the ultrasound will be performed from outside of her belly, and will show much more detail, as your developing child begins to look more and more like . . . well . . . like she's got an iguana in there or something.

An ultrasound later in the pregnancy will also reveal many recognizable organs, including that special organ that might determine whether you need to buy blue paint, or pink paint. You both will need to decide beforehand if you want to know or not. It is not an easy decision. But many couples decide to wait until the baby is born to discover its gender - going the more traditional route - and settling for yellow or light green paint.

You may wish to let your doctor and your ultrasound technician know if you don't want to find out the gender of your baby. Then you'll just have to hope that they don't slip and say,

> *"Well, we won't tell you what it is, but it sure is an*

attractive fetus, isn't she?"

Sex

(Also, See Chapter 3. Sex)

Question: *She is eight- months pregnant, can we still have sex?*

Answer: During the majority of the pregnancy, you should be able to proceed normally with your sexual activity. However, at this stage of pregnancy, it is important to remember that her body has changed (although you should never admit it), and therefore, she may not be physically able to engage in certain sexual activities (that will not be discussed here - because this is not that kind of book).

So don't hold it against her (no pun intended). Be patient, and understand that the situation is temporary, and that she probably doesn't like it any more than you do.

Probably even less.

The bottom-line to remember is to always check with the doctor for any questions regarding this issue. And don't think the doctor might be uneasy talking about sexually related topics. After all, if your doctor is an obstetrician and/or gynecologist, it is likely that she or he has had to deal with certain yeast infections all day long.

A discussion about simple sex might be refreshing.

Question: *She flipped out recently when I asked her if she thought our sex life would be the same after the baby was born. Was this not a good thing to ask?*

Answer: Asking her about it was not wrong, but it may have triggered some anxiety which she is feeling about the whole sexual situation.

Many women are concerned about the physical effects that childbirth may have on their bodies. For example, she may have fears about the endurance of her organs. Simply picturing the baby passing through the birth canal can cause women and men alike to cringe. However, these organs are typically resilient, and will often whip back in to shape, and wind up "as good as new" after delivery.

And while she probably knows this, you may have struck a nerve just by bringing up the topic.

So you might try to assure her that you will love her no matter what, and that your sex life can overcome all obstacles.

This approach may achieve better results than the rational argument of: "hey, if I was man enough to give you a good kid, than you ought to be woman enough to give me good sex." If this is really your attitude (and it is certainly your prerogative, Mr. Cro-Magnon) you really need to consider how a few well chosen cuts and stitches might affect ***your*** whole libido situation.

Also, one issue that you both should prepare for is that you may not have the time, nor the energy, for sex after the baby arrives anyway. In fact, you may find that many, if most other activities are bumped to manage the whole baby situation. So sexual concerns are not unique in this regard, it is just that the sex thing seems to stand out a little bit more than the others. (No pun intended.)

Question: *How long after the baby is born will we have to wait before we can have sexual intercourse again?*

Answer: This will be determined by your doctor, but in most cases, it will be approximately six weeks. In cases of an episiotomy or C-section, the incisions will have to heal before any activity can take place. Afterward, it will simply be a matter of physical and mental readiness.

So, try not to be pushy, nasty, moody, aggressive, spiteful or insensitive about this issue.

Because, remember, she may have, or just have had stitches. And although the sutures may have been absorbable, they were still stitches.

Alternatively, she may have received staples - a prospect that even in oz, would cause the most courageous to dread.

Incisions, stitches and staples, oh my!

In a rather sensitive place.

Which again brings to mind an important lesson learned in Chapter 10:

> *"The best thing about pregnancy is that it only occurs in women."*

Finally, as hard as it may be to believe, if she does have a decrease in sexual interest after delivery, it may have little to do with physical problems. The fact is, it could be several months afterwards before she is able to mentally accommodate this whole new baby situation into her life. Think of it this way, before she was pregnant, she may have been so busy that she had no time. Now, if you add the motherly responsibility of a new child, she has less than no time.

She has entered the new baby, time warp continuum.

So her mind maybe focused on something other than your amazing body.

Hard to believe.

Chapter 13: What to know about Month #9

"These two individuals are in charge, and it's about time you started doing what they say, when they say it."

Question: *She has been expecting for about nine months. She looks like her uterus is housing a large, if not two, watermelons. She is sleepy, fatigued, bloated, and has heartburn and indigestion. She has less nausea, and less salivation and urination. However, her breasts continue to get larger. She continues to have acne, colored stretch marks on her belly, varicose veins, nasal congestion, nosebleeds, stuffy ears, bleeding gums, swelling of her arms and legs, darkening of the skin of her face and abdomen, belly pain, backache, and leg cramps. Her belly "itches." She complains of clumsiness, loss of balance, false labor pains, leaky breasts, shortness of breath, a really fast heart rate, hemorrhoids and an exploding navel. Now she has really bad pain in the pelvic, hip, and buttock's region, and she can't even walk up or down stairs. She has so much difficulty rising from a chair that I'm thinking about renting a crane.*

I have taken your advice from the beginning, and have never admitted that I have noticed any change in her whatsoever. But there is no longer any way that I can avoid the obvious without losing any remaining portion of my credibility. She wants me to honestly tell her what I think about her appearance. I'm going to tell her the truth. What do I say?

Answer: Credibility? ***She*** is getting ready to deliver a baby, and ***you're*** worried about ***your*** credibility? Have you learned nothing? No one cares about your credibility at this point. You must continue to resist all temptation to state the obvious. The fact is, she has known you were lying since Month #1. So to change your story now would be a major strategic mistake.

And besides, at this point, there's a good chance she really doesn't care anymore.

PRE-DELIVERY ACTIVITIES

Question: *Our hospital is offering a tour of the "birthing suite." What's the difference between a "birthing suite" and a "hospital room?"*

Answer:: A whole lot, mister. Take the tour. Nothing you've ever seen in your time on this earth can prepare you for the birthing suite. It's like a Shangri-la - a Valhalla whose sole function is to facilitate the birth of your child.

It's really more like a very expensive hotel room than a hospital room. Your hospital will offer you several different choices of suites, which you will, of course, be charged for accordingly.

Try to get the one with the hot tub, if you can afford it.

It will be tastefully decorated, and will include a special bed for her and a special foldout sofa or cot for you. It may also have several comfortable chairs for any other spectators who may be around.

The TV will be neatly set in a nice wood cabinet, with all of the channels - not just one of those tiny hospital TVs that only show reruns of "Dukes of Hazard."

It'll also have its own computer to track the progress of the labor, and an overhead spotlight to help those involved to see better. Why you might even think she's giving birth at a MegaDeth concert.

Yes, the birthing suite is really just a hospital room that's been gussied up in order to make everything run a little smoother, and to attract that lucrative insurance money. But someone put a lot of time and energy into making it nice. So enjoy it while you can. Because you can bet that within an hour or so after delivery, they will probably boot your butts out of there to make room for the next panicky family.

You will then be moved to a more normal hospital room - smell, discomfort, and all.

So plan on having the resonant glow of your time in the birthing suite stay with you for many days, and weeks to come. Think of it as a vacation memory that you and she can share for a lifetime - like Disneyland, albeit a lot more expensive. On the plus side, however, remember that most insurances don't cover amusement parks. But on the other hand, Disneyland doesn't have a deductible.

CHAPTER 13: Month # 9

Question:: *One of my best friends is having his bachelor party one week before our due date. Should I go?*

Answer:: That is a decision that is likely entirely out of your hands, big boy.

Bachelor parties, by their very nature, are designed and constructed for the sole purpose of agitating the wives of the married men who are attending the party. In fact, "married" guys shouldn't even be invited to a "bachelor" party.

But somehow we always are.

And so, considering right off the top that the ***setting*** of this conflict is already lousy, the ***timing*** could probably not be any worse. The possibility of disaster looms heavy over this entire little scene, so make it a point to tread lightly, and expect to be disappointed.

If she says no, deal with it.

If she says yes, it is unlikely you will enjoy yourself anyway. You'll probably just sit there like you always do. In one room, some pitiful low-rent stripper is trying her best to get somebody's attention, while her 300-pound hairy boss-woman stands looming in the background. In the other room, video stag films show very silly people doing very silly things. Finally, you, and most of your buddies, find yourselves in the main room watching the same football game you could have watched at home.

And when you get home, she will badger you over and over as to what happened, and why you enjoy going to such things. You will then have to make up some lie, with the intent to avoid explaining what really happened, to avoid explaining how really pathetic the situation was, and to avoid explaining that you probably would have had a better time with her at home.

She can never know.

PREPARATION FOR DELIVERY

***Question:**: Should I make plans to miss a great deal of work around our due date?*

Answer:: This will depend on how many folks you can have around to lend a hand. If it's just you and she, you may want to try to have two weeks vacation or personal time, which can be flexible depending on when she starts going into labor.

Of course, most people don't have employers that will be that flexible. And can you really blame them?

They're corporate big wigs. You're nobody.

CHAPTER 13: Month # 9

You're being oppressed!

Unless labor is to be induced on a specific day, you really won't have any idea when to leave work, and when you'll be coming back. It could make things tricky.

If you have a "family support structure" that will allow her mom or aunt or whoever to be around for a week or so during the day while you go to work, then you've got a good thing. Make sure to let all those involved know how much you appreciate their diligent efforts. A good way of expressing your appreciation would be to invite them to babysit when the two of you go out for your anniversary in a few months.

And one last thing . . .

You'll be amazed, once you actually have the baby, how nice everyone will be to you. It kind of makes you wonder what was wrong with you before you had the baby.

It's kind of like, all of a sudden, you're interesting or something.

Question: *I've heard about doctors inducing labor. What is this all about?*

Answer: In many cases, her doctor will decide that it is time for the baby to be born, no matter how mother and baby feel about it.

This is how it works.

Toward the end of her pregnancy, she will probably be visiting her doctor at least once per week. During one of these visits, circumstances may arise in which her doctor may advise that labor be induced. This determination will be made for a number of different reasons, the most likely one being that the induction will benefit the health and well being of both mother and child. She may be three or four weeks away from her due date, or several weeks past it. Trust the doctor, and understand that when the doctor says it's time, ***it's time!***

The only thing about induction which could be viewed as negative is the fact that it will often take some of the excitement and drama out of the baby's birth. We all grow up with the TV-conjured idea of the little Mrs. waking up hubby in the middle of the night and of him stumbling around like an idiot in his pajamas and racing out to the car and realizing he left his wife in the house. While this may happen in some shape or form to those whose labor is not induced, it is pretty far removed from the way an induced-labor delivery will go down.

If she is to be induced, then you can methodically, drive your partner to the hospital, have her admitted to the birthing suite, and calmly wait for the doctor to light this firecracker, and let the festivities begin.

CHAPTER 13: Month # 9

Question:: *Can I demand that labor be induced on a specific day?*

Answer:: No.

Question:: *Can she?*

Answer: Yes . . . no . . . well kinda.

The decision to induce labor is based on a multitude of medical-type information. So for the non-medically-employed person, it's not a matter of how loud you can whine, or stomp your feet. In this case, your baby and your doctor agree about one major thing - they don't care about your schedule, or your anxiety, or her discomfort, or anything else that you think is so important.

These two individuals are in charge, and it's about time you started doing what they say, when they say it.

If you are a non-medical-employed person, attempts to change this is power structure is futile.

Remember. They're medical big wigs. You're nobody.

You're being oppressed!

Even if she was three weeks overdue, and was unable to move without the help of a crew of roadies to wheel her around, it's only time when the ***doctor*** says it's time. Yes, she could try to cry at the top her lungs:

> *"My dad owns this hospital!"*

And:

> *"If you people don't get this baby out of me right now, my dad is going to personally fire each and every one of you."*

But that probably won't work. Doctors are trained to deal with vapid, psychotic, overdue women and their bogus claims and threats.

However, if you are a medically-employed woman, such as a pushy woman nurse, or an aggressive woman doctor, and the baby has not arrived by the due date, it is amazing to find the sudden flexibility in the timing of induction of labor. With current induction techniques, if she is a medically-employed/connected woman, and she is much beyond her due date, she might be able to use her "connections" to literally schedule the exact time of delivery at her choosing.

You may probably hear such an individual say, "I'm going to go to the hospital next Tuesday at noon to have my baby."

And if the gender of the baby was known (quite likely because a pushy medically-employed/connected woman probably has already had ultrasounds about once a month) you may even hear her say, "I'm going to go to the hospital next Tuesday at noon to have my baby boy, and his name is going to be Brutus Winston Daniels III and his hobbies are going to be spelunking and lawn darts . . . "

But induction of labor is only an option if the baby does not decide to come before the due date.

The point is, when it comes to non-induced, spontaneous labor, the baby is the great equalizer. Because it couldn't care less about the whole medical/non-medical employment situation.

To your baby, no one is a big wig. Everyone is a nobody.

Everyone's oppressed!

LABOR AND GETTING TO THE HOSPITAL

Question:: *Is it possible that she could go into labor without breaking her water?*

Answer:: Yes.

And it is more likely than you may think. So while the release of amniotic fluid is often the sign that labor has started, many women will begin labor with other symptoms.

In fact, she may not break her water until she is sitting on your new leather car seats on the way to the hospital, or until you are standing at the check-in desk at the hospital.

You just never know.

Question: *How long after her water breaks will she have the baby?*

Answer: Water breaking is no harbinger as to the duration of her labor. Plenty of women have their babies minutes after their water breaks, while just as many others are just at the beginning of a thirty-hour journey into pure hell.

Which again brings to mind an important lesson learned in Chapter 10:

> *"The best thing about pregnancy is that it only occurs in women."*

Question: *Will it be necessary for me to drive her straight to the hospital once her water breaks?*

Answer: The first thing you should do after her water breaks, aside from getting some paper towels, is to get her doctor on the phone. During this conversation (that will undoubtedly be somewhere between 11:00 P.M. and 5:00 A.M.), you will finally understand why her doctor gets paid so much. The doctor will calm and soothe you at a time when all of your nerve endings are crackling and sizzling, and you feel as if you've never been more helpless.

Her doctor will then ask a series of questions, and then decide what the next course of action should be. As a general rule, it is best not to scream, curse, or hiss at the doctor. If you cannot help yourself, her doctor will probably understand, and adjust your bill accordingly.

Remain calm. In many cases, the doctor may decide to have you wait at home, even if her water has broken, until there are more signs that she needs to be taken to the hospital.

In the event the doctor tells you to wait at home for a while, and she is writhing in agony, telling you that there's no possible way that she can wait any longer, then just call the doctor back . . .

Put her on the phone . . .

You start the car.

Question: *Will it be necessary to drive like a maniac to get to the hospital?*

Answer: Hopefully not. The time frame with which you will be working may not necessitate a "Starsky and Hutch" type ride to the hospital. If you find your car tipped up on two wheels while going around corners, you may be pushing it a little bit.

Yes, the temptation exists to use the impending birth as an excuse to break a few laws. But be careful. Certain police departments in certain areas of the country may not be as ***cooperative*** as those in other areas. So thinking you might scam your way out of a speeding ticket, or perhaps a severe beating, may not be as plausible as you may think.

It is important to have several routes planned out in advance. If you need to drive on an interstate to get there, decide what you'll do if the interstate is closed or backed up. If you plan to use residential streets, allow for traffic lights, rush hour congestion, school bus hours or any other difficulties which may impede your journey.

You may need to make special considerations if you:

* Live in a rural area and will have a relatively long trip to get to the hospital.

* Live in a large city and don't have a car, thereby creating the need to use public transportation or cabs to get to the hospitals.

* Are Amish and will be using a horse-and-buggy to get to the hospital.

But even with your best plans, there is a good chance that when she goes into labor, you won't be there. In this case, you will have to just meet her at the hospital while someone else drives her to the hospital - like one of her parents, or a friend, or perhaps your seventeen-year-old neighbor who just got his license

He'll get her there in a hurry!

***Question:**: Once we arrive at the hospital, when and where do we meet the team of physicians who will rush out to meet us at the car, throw her on the stretcher, and immediately wheel her down to the labor and delivery area?*

Answer: Hold on there Mr. ER. You are living in TV fantasy land - not reality.

The fact is, it is unlikely that anyone will meet you at your car. You are going to have to drive up to the labor and delivery area of the hospital, and walk in the hospital just like you were going to have a bunion removed or something. And unless your baby's head is literally winking at you out of the womb, it is likely your first stop will probably be the check-in desk. Here, you will need to register, and give the most crucial medical information required during the whole pregnancy situation . . .

Her insurance card.

Afterwards, you and she can leisurely go to the labor and delivery area while sweat is pouring off your head, and her water is flowing from between her legs.

What a Kodak moment.

Chapter 14: What to know during the whole labor and delivery situation

"We have all certainly heard that line enough to know it is never to be taken seriously."

BEFORE LABOR ACTIVITY

Question: *We attended a class on pain relief, but I'm still not clear on the epidural. Should she get an epidural? When should she ask for an epidural? What is an epidural?*

Answer: Inside the bones of the back is the spinal cord, which carries nerves such as her pain fibers. The epidural region is next to the spinal cord. Epidural anesthesia is when numbing medicine is administered between the backbones, into the epidural region, around the spinal cord.

It numbs the nerves.

Once she receives the epidural anesthesia, she will be mostly numb from the waist down, and be able to experience the birth of her child, free of pain.

That's the theory, anyway.

However, she might be a little leery in view of all the stories about how her friend's epidural "wore off" or "fell out." Stephen King could not have described anything more frightening.

But even though epidural anesthesia is the "drug" of choice for most women, many experts (including some of the more militant women's groups) warn that epidural anesthesia has many potentially serious short, and long term side effects.

But, because you are a man, you may not be particularly persuaded. But the facts suggest (as opposed to what you might otherwise expect from such groups) that these potential concerns are quite real.

So, hopefully, she has already thought about it, and decided whether or not she wanted to take such a risk, ***long before*** she got to the hospital.

Partially due to the potential risks of the epidural, plenty of women still prefer natural child birth, i.e., without drugs. And if these women have a room down the hall from you, you'll know it by the terrified moans and shrieks careening down the hallway.

And you thought your hangnail was painful.

Even the most committed woman desiring "natural childbirth," may eventually choose a different path once the baby's head has pried her cervix open about six centimeters. She may suddenly find that the person she most wants in the delivery room is no longer her doctor, her mother, or even you.

Suddenly, the anesthesiologist may become the most important person in her life.

This is natural. It also seems normal.

Which brings us to the "tip of the day."

The following piece of advice will finally make you seem sensitive to her, and brilliant to her family and friends. And best of all, the advice is both practical and logical.

And the advice is this:

> *If, after weighing all the risks and benefits, she has decided she definitely chooses drugs during labor, ask the nurse and/or anesthesiologist to start the epidural at the first hint of pain and/or the earliest it is thought to be safe.*

Many practical concerns support this recommendation.

First of all, if she has decided that she definitely wants the epidural anesthesia at some point, then why wait? What is the benefit?

Secondly, if labor has truly started, and the pain has started, it ain't going to get better. It will only get worse. Again, no need to wait.

Finally, seizing the earliest opportunity to start the epidural avoids potential long delays later. For example, suppose the friendly anesthesiologist visits the room and asks if she wants to have the epidural started (which involves placing an access port in the back region.). Suppose she wants to act brave and declines because she is only experiencing moderate pain right now. The anesthesiologist then leaves to care for fifteen other women who just hit the hospital ready to deliver. (Believe it, it ***can*** happen. It ***does*** happen.) Now it may be hours before the anesthesiologist may be able to return, regardless of how much pain she has.

These are hours of suffering that did not have to happen. And guess who will be expected to take responsibility for her pain?

But now suppose you were smart enough to read this book. So instead, she took your advice, and requested the epidural sooner rather than later. And when the pain worsened, all someone had to do was simply turn up the drip.

No other assembly required.

And the rest of the whole delivery experience is just a walk on the beach - all because of your brilliant advice.

You have just become a credit to your gender.

Question: *Is there any limit to the amount of people in the birthing suite while she is in labor?*

Answer:: That would be up to individual hospital policy, but the best advice would be to limit the number to the barest minimum. There are only so many players that should be involved with this particular game.

The two of you should mutually decide, in advance, who gets to be in the room itself, and who really would be ***much*** more comfortable in the waiting room.

Because it is not unheard of for a woman in labor to have a

steady flow of visitors in and out of the birthing suite for hours on end. And while she may not be in a great deal of pain in the beginning, she may not be feeling much like "entertaining" extended family members while wearing a gown that ties in the back.

Oh, she may be smiling and kissy huggy while everyone's parading by her stirrup-studded delivery gurney, giving her chocolate, and asking "how are you feeling" for crying out loud. But deep inside she's seething and wishing you'd get all of these people the hell out of here - now!

So assign a family member as your liaison to the rest of your family and close friends. Ask this person to be a buffer between you and them, conveying information, progress reports, etcetera. (A prior employment as a bar bouncer is the type of person you are looking for). Put this person in charge of making necessary phone calls and acting as a "gofer" in the event that you need anything outside of the hospital.

It might be advisable to pay this person an hourly salary.

An alternative, practical way to handle this is to have your doctors and nurses serve as "bad guy" if you want them too, and shoo certain individuals out of the room.

Just be sure that they don't shoo you out too, especially if the only other place left to go is with the rest of the family, and away from the football game on the birthing suite television.

CHAPTER 14: During Labor and Delivery

Question: *I don't want to be there during the delivery. I don't think she even wants me there. I think it might make me sick. How do I get out of this?*

Answer: Not long ago, delivery at most hospitals was witnessed only by doctors and nurses, with an occasional grandmother there occasionally for moral support. Panicky dads were left in the waiting room, walled-in like veal in a fattening crate.

My, how times have changed.

Now dads are expected to be there for every second of it. And regardless of how you feel about it, you are suppose to be there pal, and you can't weasel out of it. Remember the lesson from Chapter 12:

> *"Your level of caring is defined by how willing you are to endure experiences out of your element. And the more painful the experience, the greater your demonstration of caring."*

And don't be fooled by her statement that:

> *"You don't have to be there if you don't want to be."*

We have all certainly heard that line enough to know it is never to be taken seriously.

Question: *Would it be improper if I left during her labor to get a breather, or a cup of coffee?*

Answer: Most likely not, but you may want to ask first. Don't just say, "Okay, I'll be back shortly," and scamper out of there.

Yes, everyone will need a break. And there may be some down time when you could disappear for twenty minutes or so. Bring a pager or cell phone if you have one, or stay close enough to her room that someone can retrieve you if needed.

Because if you miss the event . . .

If she absolutely refuses to let you leave, just give in. Someone else can bring you coffee. Stay with her, because she probably really needs you.

And don't be fooled by her statement that:

> *"You don't have to stay here if you don't want to."*

As noted before, we have all certainly heard that line enough to know it is never to be taken seriously. And it's not going to be worth the time or energy to find out if she really means it or not.

So do what she says now. And keep a list. That way, you can remind her about it later whenever you get tagged that ill-deserved "insensitive" label again.

Pay backs are hell!

CHAPTER 14: During Labor and Delivery

DURING LABOR ACTIVITY

Question: *Now that I am stuck during the whole delivery situation, what am I up against?*

Answer: Delivery is a montage of blood, mucus, and screams of agony . . . you know . . . the kinds of things you would expect from such an ageless miracle.

So you need to be prepared. Some fathers perceive this experience with wonder and excitement, and want to participate as much as possible.

Others just pass out.

If you get sick, that's O.K. It happens a lot. Let's face it, as great a wonderment as it may be, the birth of a child is one of the most gruesome biological processes imaginable. So if you find yourself the least bit lightheaded, don't stand up. And if you know you're turning pale, and the nurse asks you how you are doing, tell her the truth. Failure to admit that you've got a problem will only make things worse.

For example, admitting that you are a little queasy, and staying in your seat instead of standing to fully view the whole delivery situation will soon be forgotten. However, if you faint and fall face first into a hemorrhaging womb . . .

It ***will*** be remembered.

Question: *We have been told that active labor may last for hours. During that time, it doesn't seem like much else is going on except for shrieks of pain that make it difficult to hear the televised college football game of the week. When the nurse comes in the room and turns down the volume, is it O.K. if I turn it back up when she leaves?*

Answer: Hey, it's your prerogative, Mr. Cro-Magnon. However, remember that most nurses are still women. And as unfair as it may seem, they may be more inclined to be concerned with your partner's active labor, than whether or not you get to see the end of the Alabama/Auburn game.

Question: *I've seen a million TV shows where the woman is having a baby, and the father is yelling at the woman to breathe a certain way. She then takes deep breaths, and whooshes it out through her mouth and nose. Suddenly, she seems to have a substantial relief of pain.*

They didn't go over this in our prenatal classes. Why?

Answer: Certain breathing techniques are said to alleviate pain during child birth.

CHAPTER 14: During Labor and Delivery

"Hee Hee! Hoo Hoo!"

One can only imagine that this was the response immediately after someone suggested that deep breathing could relieve the pain during childbirth.

"Hee Hee! Hoo Hoo!"

So, while it is true that women who deliver using natural childbirth methods, without pain-relieving medicine, do a lot of breathing . . .

They also do a lot of screaming.

This is natural. ***This*** is normal.

Question: *I've seen a million TV shows where the woman is having a baby, and yelling at the man, cursing the man, slapping the man, and screaming that the pain experienced during the whole delivery situation is solely, and completely, the man's fault. But I don't think this is anything I have to worry about because she never curses, and is basically a rational person. So, in my case, when she is at the peak of pain, and sweat is dripping from every pore of her body, will I really have to be prepared about foul language?*

Will I really have to worry about bodily injury?

Answer: Yes.

Be prepared for some very colorful language, and perhaps some words you've never heard before.

And you'd better wear a cup.

Question: *The doctors and nurses just asked us if it was O.K. if a medical student watched the delivery. She asks me what I think. I just don't know. What do I say?*

Answer: This is a decision that should be left totally up to her. Soon she will have countless strangers examining, poking, surveying, and generally reviewing the most intimate, private parts of her physical self. So on the one hand, one more person won't have much practical impact on the most undignified situation that anyone could be put through. On the other hand, one more person may be just one more person too many.

So if she is the least uncomfortable about it, just say no.

Medical science will survive.

Question: *What is the umbilical cord, and will I get to cut it? And what is that placenta thing anyway?*

Answer: The uterus (otherwise known as the womb) is an organ in the pelvic region of the woman that looks like a balloon with really fat walls. At the bottom is the round opening ("cervical os" or cervical opening). During regular menstruation (before pregnancy), the first weeks are dedicated toward building up the inside wall of the uterus. The last week is dedicated toward tearing it down. The tearing down of the inside wall of the uterus (with the monthly debris coming out of the uterus, through the cervical opening, and out the vagina) is the dreaded "bleeding" that we have all heard so much about.

At the top of the uterus are two ducts (fallopian tubes) that come from the ovaries (that contain the eggs). Once a month, if the ovaries cooperate, the egg is released from one of the ovaries, goes through the fallopian duct/tube, and is delivered into the inside cavity of the uterus. If at the same time, millions of your sperm just happened to have been swimming by, by route of the cervical opening, and also entered into the cavity of the uterus, then one of them may penetrate and "fertilize" the egg. If this fertilization occurs, then the egg may stick ("implant") on the inside wall of the uterus and grow. As this process continues, the structure that remains attached to the uterus becomes thick and round and is known as the placenta. The tube from the placenta to the fetus is known as the umbilical cord.

The whole point of all of this is to allow stuff in her blood (like nutrients) to go to the uterus, where the placenta decides which of the stuff continues on to the fetus. If the placenta thinks it's O.K., then the stuff goes on through the placenta, through the umbilical cord, onto the fetus through the connection at the fetus's navel.

This is the way it works during the whole pregnancy situation.

However, at delivery the baby won't be fed through its navel ("belly button") anymore. So the umbilical cord and placenta aren't needed, and have to go.

That is why, immediately after birth, the umbilical cord is "clamped," thereby stopping the flow of blood. After it is clamped, it is usually cut.

But who ***gets*** to cut it?

Individual hospitals differ in their policies concerning this practice. Some may not consider it worth the risk to put a sharp object in a new father's hand. So while it has been said that it is good luck for the father to do this, if you screw it up, or if you pass out, then perhaps it wasn't so lucky.

So if you don't ***get*** to cut the cord, don't worry. You'll have plenty of other stuff to occupy your interest.

After the whole umbilical cord cutting situation, the placenta is still hanging in there like a useless relative, and has got to go. Because it is still attached to the umbilical cord, it is likely that you will see the doctor slightly pulling on the cord, while massaging the abdomen in order to deliver the placenta. But, as much as everyone would like to speed the process up, it is unlikely that your doctor will become so impatient that he or she starts yanking on the cord to jerk it off the inside lining of the uterus.

So relax.

Remember. The delivery of all the stuff left over after the delivery ("afterbirth") is a natural process. Unless a problem arises, the whole afterbirth situation should be allowed to happen naturally.

Question: *How soon after the baby is born will I get to hold it?*

Answer: Many factors will go into determining this. In the case of a normal delivery, the baby will be taken directly to a scale, weighed and cleaned and then handed directly to the parents. You'll be holding your bambino in a matter of minutes.

If complications arise (involving mother, baby, or both) this entire situation could be completely different. Don't worry too much if they take mother or baby away. Just ask a doctor or nurse to be straight with you and tell you exactly what's going on. They will most likely tell you. Try to be prepared for any eventuality, as difficult as that might sound. Remember that the hospital staff is taking every step to make sure that the health and safety of all persons involved in the delivery are maintained.

Question: *I've heard about babies looking slimy and shriveled-up when they are born. Is that true?*

Answer: Yes. Your baby has been living for the last nine months inside of a womb, which is a self-contained unit where food, waste materials, and all other matters of nastiness are sloshing around. Suddenly, the baby is forced out this little cubby, and it's just natural to assume that the little cherub will emerge with some of this goo still covering its skin.

Don't worry. It washes off.

And when the nurses hand you your baby, it will likely be a rosy-red little skin-bundle with bug-eyes and a mewling little mouth.

It will also be the most perfect thing you've ever seen - goo and all.

And it will be even more perfect if it's handed to you in a towel.

Question: *We want to video tape the delivery. I plan to take the home video camera, and crouch behind the doctor to get a great close up as the matted, hairy head of our newborn is pushing through my wife's bloody vagina.*

Some of my friends have expressed little enthusiasm toward receiving copies of this video.

Others think this is just weird.

Is this weird?

Answer: Yes.

This is entirely too weird.

Look, if you just ***have*** to video tape the whole morbid delivery situation, and you want it to be suitable for others, then at least consider avoiding action shots of her pelvic region. Nothing will be lost if you, and your video camera, stay at the head of the bed as the intact baby is first revealed by the doctor raising the child above the sheets of privacy.

And in this way, you don't have to worry about video rating systems, or V-chips.

SPECIAL LABOR ACTIVITY

Question: *One of her sisters had to be induced with a pitocin drip. What is this?*

Answer: If the pregnancy is not progressing as quickly as the doctor would like, a pitocin (oxytocin) "drip" in the veins may be started. Pitocin is a hormone (that the body already makes) that causes the muscles of the uterus to contract.

Think of pitocin as a very demanding personal trainer for her uterus.

The intent is to cause the uterus to flex to the point that it blasts the reluctant kid out. This is usually done only if a medical problem requires it, if your bundle of joy is just being too pigheaded to come out on time, or if the doctor has somewhere else to go.

Question: *What is a breach birth?*

Answer: A breach birth occurs when the position of the baby is reversed in the birth canal, so that the feet are ready to come out first instead of the head. This occurs in humans, as well as with many other mammals. The positioning can often be corrected by the doctor (or the veterinarian) by moving the unborn around before delivery. If this is unsuccessful, the doctor may discuss, beforehand, the relative risks and benefits of caesarian section, versus delivering the baby feet first.

And remember, as the day of delivery gets closer and closer, don't be surprised if the baby finally gets its head together in the right position, right before delivery. (You should be so lucky.)

One could speculate that this is a way to add just one more worry to already anxious parents.

So don't be too concerned about breach births. Doctors and nurses are prepared for almost any eventuality involving childbirth, so once you've made it to the maternity ward, remain calm and let them do their jobs.

Question: *I've heard that a lot of women will have to have their baby delivered by cesarian section. How does this work?*

Answer: A C-Section is a procedure named after Caesar who was stabbed. Hence, a C-Section involves an incision with a knife made in the mother's abdomen, through which the baby is removed from the womb. The incision can be vertical (from the navel to the pelvis), or it may be low and horizontal, four to five inches long, and is called a "bikini cut."

Either one may leave a scar. But, on the one hand, the "bikini scar" may be less noticeable in the long run. But on the other hand, at this point, wearing a bikini will probably be the last thing on her mind.

Question: *I've been preparing myself to watch the birth of my child, but I'm wondering if I will have to watch the delivery if she needs to have a C-Section. Will I really have to go through that?*

Answer: Most likely, unless you insist on seeing it, the actual surgical procedure involving the C-Section will be hidden from you. The mother will be moved to an operating room, where all preparations, and quite often, the incision itself will be completed. Afterwards, you will be brought into the room. You will remain close to your partner's head, encouraging her that all is well, while they lovingly yank your new born offspring right out of her belly!

Don't worry, she'll be heavily anesthetized, and won't feel a thing. Once the anesthesia wears off, she may experience some pain, and she will most likely be quite sore for a while after the procedure.

And the pain is very real. It is so real that even most insurance companies allow a little extra time in the hospital.

So you know it' s ***got*** to be real.

CHAPTER 15: What to know after the whole delivery situation

"You are in more trouble than you can ever know."

AFTER THE WHOLE DELIVERY SITUATION

Question: *Will the baby be able to sleep with us in our hospital room the first night?*

Answer: Yes, many hospitals will allow the baby to sleep in the hospital room with you on the first night, depending on the condition of the baby. But don't feel bad if both you and her find a reason why that it might be "best for the baby" to spend the first night in the nursery.

You, and it, ***will*** need the rest.

Besides, if mom's asleep, most hospitals will take the baby back to the nursery anyway. And when mom awakes, the baby can be easily ordered back to the room anytime.

It's kind of like room service - except with more limited choices.

Question: *Will the hospital staff ask us for the baby's name right away?*

Answer: No. Once the baby is born, it will be identified by its gender and its last name only. Its nursery bed will have this information on a card attached to it, along with the date of birth and the child's weight.

The baby may also have an identifying band around some appendage with the same identification number or name as the band that will be placed around the parents' wrist.

It is all a matter of security.

Nevertheless, even though a last name and a number are all that the hospital requires, you'd better have that name picked out already - because everyone's going to start asking you right away what it is. Furthermore, if your partner is unconscious following the delivery, make sure you give the correct name. Because if she wakes up and finds out that you've told the world that your new baby girl's name is Catherine with a "C" rather than Katherine with a "K," you are in big trouble, buddy.

Finally, it is generally not a good idea to inform her within 24 hours after delivery that you really don't like the name that you and she had already chosen. Because, if you unilaterally decide to change the whole baby name situation, you may find that she responds with the same colorful language you heard during the whole delivery situation.

Question: *When will the hospital take the baby's picture?*

Answer: Many times, a picture of the newborn will be taken by a hospital photographer, usually in the nursery before the baby goes home. If you want them (and she will), you can choose anywhere from a single picture to an entire package of different sizes of pictures. And, not too surprising, she will probably want them all.

Question: *Will the baby's footprints be taken right away?*

Answer: No. The foot-printing procedure takes place in the nursery following delivery. The baby will be cleaned, diapered, foot printed, filtered, lubed, tucked, channeled, lowered and louvered.

You will, of course, be charged accordingly for this service.

Question: *How long will it take until our family and friends are able to see the baby?*

Answer: Most procedures in the nursery are usually complete, barring any complications, an hour or two after the delivery. Loved ones will be able to see the baby behind the glass windows of the nursery.

CHAPTER 15: After the delivery

Just like in the movies.

Just like a slab of salmon at the grocery store.

It never fails to bring a tear.

Once the baby is brought to the mother's hospital room, visitors will probably be allowed to come in and hold the baby. Different hospitals will have different policies regarding visitors, so be aware of that. And although these policies and rules may seem excessive, remember, they are in the best interest of the child. Because you never know when Uncle Fester, with a bad case of tuberculosis and several open skin sores wants to play huggie face with your new child.

Banning his participation in the whole new baby situation can easily, and conveniently, be blamed on the whole hospital "policy" situation.

Question: *She has just delivered. Is giving out cigars still the thing to do?*

Answer: If you smoke 'em, yes. If you don't, maybe no.

But if giving cigars is a thing for you, then look to the newly created grandparents.

In fact, ***always*** look to the grandparents.

Grandparents should be thought of as an endless source of help, emotional support, and money. So have them hook you up on the cigars. Because no matter what you may think of their abilities now, you will soon become amazed at their wealth of practical knowledge - even to the point of being astounded at their ability to find a box of cigars with the appropriate "It's a Boy" or "It's a Girl" on the plastic wrapper.

And insist on real cigars. It's a time-honored tradition that will make you feel wonderful, no matter how politically incorrect it is. Unfortunately, if you're a control freak who likes to have everything handled ahead of time, you won't be able to get the cigars in advance unless you already know what gender your baby is going to be.

This is where "Grandpa" comes in. Dispatch him from the hospital to "Crazy Joe's Tobacco Hut," and he'll be thrilled to be sent on such a mission.

And don't send him to find them in the hospital gift shop. They will probably only stock chocolate cigars, because chocolate is ***so*** much healthier than tobacco. If they do carry real cigars, they'll probably be stale, and priced way too high. The hospital gift shop will have plenty of overpriced junk just waiting to be sold to a gushing new dad (sucker) like you.

If you work it right, you'll never have to set a foot in the gift shop, nor will you have to prepare a meal for the next few weeks. Your parents, or her parents will appreciate being given a job to do, and will do it well. Most likely, they have been waiting a long time for this moment, so let them get excited and participate in the festivities.

And this may be the perfect opportunity to patch things up with them after the doctors and nurses ran them out of the birthing suite - at your request.

Question: *I've seen wooden stork signs on people's front yards announcing the name and weight of the baby. Do I have to do this?*

Answer: No, and you probably won't. This is the kind of sentimental commercialism that, is just perfect for the new grandparents.

Again, let them take care of all of that stuff.

Question: *About twelve hours after delivery, the family had gone, and the baby was in the nursery. As a result, we had some quiet time together in the hospital - just she and I. It was a moment of intimacy. Among the things we discussed was how emotionally upset she was about her appearance. And as I looked in those sad and tearful eyes, I could tell she was yearning for me to say something supportive. Fortunately I was prepared. I told her that I had a surprise waiting for her at home. I had already gone out and bought a collection of* *exercise equipment, membership to the YMCA, coupon to a weight loss center, and a prescription for the latest weight-loss pill.*

She didn't seem to brighten up as I would have thought. In fact, she asked me to leave so she could get some sleep. And now her mother, and the nurses, won't talk to me. Should I have kept it a surprise until we got home? Where did I do wrong this time?

Answer: You may recall that before each of the chapters of this book dealing with the months of pregnancy, you were instructed to deny that her appearance changed in any way before delivery. After delivery, it is probably best to keep the charade going for at least the next six weeks. Because about six weeks after delivery, the sympathy factor for her will be virtually nonexistent, and you can go back to being a man without the fear of being tagged with that ill-deserved "insensitive" label again. Yes, she will still get upset if you buy her items that suggest that she needs to lose weight, and tone up. But six weeks after delivery, it will just be her opinion, rather than the opinion of an entire community of women.

Question: *Several hours after delivery, nothing else much was going on. I was really tired. The hospital wasn't a very comfortable place to sleep. She said it would be O.K. if I went home. The following morning, she called me at home from the hospital to see how **I** was doing.*

CHAPTER 15: After the delivery

Do I have a great partner or what?

Answer: You are in more trouble than you can ever know.

Question: *Now that she has delivered, and all the hoopla is over, and she has a few weeks off from work, what is the best way to kick back, and enjoy the break of the next few days with our new baby.*

Answer: Break? What break? Your ordeal is just beginning. In fact the first few days after delivery can be the worst part of the whole newborn situation.

The basic problems are these.

First of all, if this is your first child, then you don't know what to expect. So anything remotely unexpected that this wrapped bundle of joy does will likely send mom into a frenzy. A wheeze becomes suffocation. A snore becomes bronchial tube obstruction. Spitting up becomes an intestinal emergency.

This is not to say that these symptoms shouldn't be taken seriously.

But it is to say that you just don't know.

Secondly, once she returns home, she may try to become the Supermom she always envisioned herself to be. And it is unlikely she will never meet her expectations. The end result is that she comes home from the hospital, after having virtually no sleep for about nine months, right after going through one of the most painful, and traumatic medical procedures known to humankind, (with or without stitches), only to have to deal with a totally helpless life-form, that constantly needs to be cleaned and fed, and is totally dependent on her for it's very survival.

But enough about dealing with you.

There's the baby too.

The baby must be fed. The baby must be changed. The baby must cry. The baby must occupy every waking, and non-waking hour of the day for the next several months.

So the point is this: you must make some arrangements so that someone is available to help manage the baby the first few days she returns from the hospital. It could be you. It could be family or friends. But you must insist that Supermom give up some of her imprinted, inborn, guilt-tainted need to do everything.

Accepting her argument that "I'm the mother, and I'm the only one who can do it" is a ticket to disaster - particularly in the first few days.

Question: *I might be just dreaming here, but I think I might just have it made with this whole new baby situation. I have offered to get up at night and feed the baby. But she wants to breast* *feed. I have offered to help change and dress the baby. But she feels this imprinted, inborn, guilt-tainted need to do everything. In every instance that I have offered to help, she has indicated that she is the mother, and is the only one who can do things right.*

So since she declined my help, and she wants to do everything, and since there is no reason in the world for both of us to lose sleep, doesn't this mean I don't have to worry about losing sleep?

Answer: Yes, you are exactly right.

You are dreaming.

Because, even if she feels she has to do everything, and even if she declines your help, that doesn't mean she doesn't resent your sleeping while she is doing all the work. Therefore, don't be surprised that when feeding time comes at 2:00 A.M., even if you live in a three-story mansion with 25 rooms, you will find that the baby must be transported to the only place the feeding process can take place, which just happens to be within a few feet of wherever you are sleeping.

And if the baby has to be changed at 2:00 A.M., then, again, the baby must be transported to the only place where the changing process can take place, which just happens to be withing a few feet of wherever you are sleeping.

The point is, while it is true that she may have declined your help, while it is true that she may have this need to do everything, and while it is true that there is no reason in the world for both of you to lose sleep, she ***will*** find a way to get you up, or keep you up along with her.

And what are you going to say?

"Get out of here. I want to sleep."

???

You're stuck.

This is not a reasonable world.

Question: *Now that she has delivered, I am looking forward to her being less emotional. How many minutes after delivery do I have to wait before things will go back to the way they were before the pregnancy?*

Answer: First of all, things will never go back the way they use to be before the pregnancy. Secondly, if you thought she was emotional ***before*** delivery, just wait until ***after*** delivery. The week or so after delivery makes premenstrual syndrome look like a picnic.

It is like PMS[3].

AFTER DELIVERY NECESSITIES

Question: *She just delivered, and is going to be in the hospital for another 24 hours, depending upon the decision of her insurance case manager. I want to everything to be set up just right when she gets home. What all do we need?*

Answer: Obviously this is largely going to depend upon your lifestyle. However, some essentials you might think about include:

I. Car seats

In most cases, it will be your responsibility to drive her, and the baby home. Many hospitals will not let you leave unless you have a car seat in your car. They don't care whether or not your car has brakes, wheels, or a windshield, but it ***must*** have a car seat. So get them immediately for your car, and her car.

And remember, car seats make great gifts to the grandparents who will likely be doing a lot of the things that you don't want to do. And buying them car seats is a minimal gesture that can only facilitate further help on their part in the future.

What a great gift idea!

And one last thing. Most car seats are for babies around eight or more pounds. If your child is smaller at birth, it probably won't fit in the car sear. Its head will flop back and forth in bizarre contortions that will scare both of you to death. So why would hospitals insist that a baby be placed in a car seat on the way home, when it seems it may actually be safer to be in the arms of the mother - who could be wearing a safety belt?

It's big brother, man.

Nevertheless, you don't want to start out the whole new baby situation arguing with the nurse about the conflict between individual liberties versus the public good. So just remember to bring plenty of towels. They can be wrapped around the baby to make a better fit in the car seat.

And the baby is safe and secure.

And the State is sustained for another day.

II. A diaper strategy.

The whole diaper situation has become one of marketing, environmental, and medical confusion. Basically, each choice has its own advantages and disadvantages.

Cloth diapers are thought to be the most environmentally safe.

If you are the "earthy" sort (wear sandals, wire-rim glasses, and have a picture of John Lennon beside the closet with the bell-bottoms you wish you could still wear), then this is probably the best option for you. Cloth diapers may also be associated with less "diaper rash" However, this advantage may be negated with the use of plastic, waterproof pants that often have to be placed over the cloth diapers to avoid the transfer of Junior's waste products to cribs, couches, adult clothing, carpets, etc. Also, the use of cloth diapers requires the development of dexterity skills in the safe use of baby pins on a squirming, often non-cooperative, screaming fruit of your loins.

Ouch!

Cloth diaper services are also available. Basically, you trade "dirty" diapers for clean ones that are delivered to your home once a week. Just be sure you understand the "rules" of your service as to how the service wants the diapers to be handled before they are picked up.

Disposable diapers are not as environmentally friendly. They are a significant contributor to land fills. Each year, over a million metric tons of wood pulp, as well as tons of non-biodegradable plastic are required to manufacture disposable diapers.

However, disposable diapers are very convenient. Basically, they, are composed of an inner paper layer, treated with chemicals to increase absorbency, all covered by an outer layer of plastic. With the easy-to-use adhesive tape, they typically are very easy to take on and off the baby. Finally, they can be discarded in a diaper pale, which contains yet another plastic trash-bag like container, for easy transfer to the trash.

Whatever your (her) choice, the plan needs to be in place before she gets home with the baby. The necessity of this urgency will become apparent within minutes after you arrive home.

And there is one last thing you should know about the whole baby diaper situation. It is likely that you ***will*** have to change the baby at some point. You can't weasel out of this one. Some fathers change the baby only if the mother is not available, and it just ***has*** to be done to avoid accusations of child abuse. (Hey, it's your prerogative, Mr. Cro-Magnon.) Some fathers change the baby more often than the mother. Most fathers are somewhere in between. But you should be aware that even if you only change the baby once for every hundred times she changes the baby, you will still experience a compelling need to announce that you performed this act. A mysterious force will require you to demand recognition for performing this single act, which she routinely performs multiple times a day, every day. If you feel uncomfortable with the lack of logic of this compulsion - relax. After the illogical, emotional, hormonal wind-tunnel she just put you through for the past nine months, you are entitled to a little expression of ridiculousness.

III. Food

If she plans on breast feeding, then skip to the section below. If not, then you will have to be prepared to bottle feed. So read on.

When you leave the hospital, it is possible that you will be given "free samples" of baby formula. Yes, this is an act of shameless promotion on the part of the baby formula industry.

But what do you care?

You got free stuff.

And you will hear a lot of noise about the different kinds of formula. And it may seem that if you make one wrong decision, then you will responsible for the starving of your baby.

Relax.

If you just accept the fact that you are going to spend ***way*** too much money on formula, then all you need to know are some basic rules.

Rule #1:

Try to find a formula that is as close to mothers' milk as possible. Running down to the market and getting "Food Mart 2% Bessie's Best Day Old Milk" on sale for $1.00 per gallon ain't going to get it done. Instead, you need to buy multiple bottles of special formulated baby formula, that will probably cost more than bottles of pure plutonium.

Rule #2:

The choice of which formula is best will depend on the recommendations of the doctor, as well as what the child will actually drink.

Rule #3:

Formula is supplied in different preparations. First of all, if you have lots of cash, cupboard space, and/or are just really lazy, then get the ready-made bottles, that, with the addition of a clean, screw-on nipple, are ready-to-go.

Or secondly, you might want to get a can of the stuff to pour. However, ***someone*** will have to clean the bottles and nipples before the formula is poured. Because not only is formula good for the growth of your child, but it is also an excellent source of nutrients for nasty disease-producing bacteria. And should you try to save time by "forgetting" to clean the bottle, or "forgetting" to get the crusted old milk out of the nipple hole, then you will lose this time tenfold when the baby is up all night crying with stomach upset, diarrhea, fever, etc.

Finally, cans or packets of powder are available. This might be the least expensive route to take. However, in this case, not only will you have to clean the bottle and nipple before use, but you will also have to mix the stuff with water by following directions. (And we know how you love following directions.)

And you need to know that the baby's mouth is not a sterile area, something you will soon realize when your little human disposal proceeds to put all sorts of nastiness in its mouth. Therefore, although mom may have the compulsive need to sterilize the planet, unless you drink from a well, or have a water supply with nasty parasites and bacteria, then it is unlikely that you really need to boil everything.

(And we know how you were so wanting to have the whole "boil some water!" situation actually mean something.)

The bottom line is that you will probably buy several of each of these formula preparations, and then use them, depending upon when convenience, or cost is the biggest priority.

Rule #4:

Ask the doctor what type of nipple is best. (We are referring to the bottle type, not hers.) The doctor will probably give a bogus answer indicating that the doctor doesn't really know. So if you want a ***real*** answer, find the nurse on your hospital floor with the most experience before you leave. In fact, after the delivery, this nurse will probably give you more practical information than any doctor.

Regardless of what nipple is recommended, you will probably have a hard time finding the exact right type or brand. So you might want to spend her last few hours in the hospital running around town finding the right kind.

If nothing else, this gives you a great excuse to get out of the boring, creepy hospital again.

Finally, even if you have gotten the exact right brand of nipples, it is likely that a good percentage of them won't work. The seal will leak. Or, most commonly, the hole will be so small that the baby will have no chance of getting any milk out of it. In this case, you will have to find some safe way to carefully, and slightly widen the hole.

Alternatively, you could ask the doctor if there's a safe way to clean and sterilize your drill bits, and use a power drill to solve the problem.

And isn't finding a way to use your electric tools again just what you have been looking forward to for a long, long time - since the beginning of this whole baby situation?

IV. Clothing

It is unlikely that this will be a problem. She, or her mom, or your mom, or some other XX chromosome type has probably already handled the whole baby clothes situation. However, it might be worth your while to at least know some of the terminology (See Glossary of "What Words to Know.")

Furthermore, if you have any relatives or friends at all, you will probably receive so many clothes that your baby will grow faster than the opportunity to wear them all.

Many of them will likely never be worn.

And best of all, not only is this factual and common, but it is also provides you a ready-made excuse if someone gives you a baby outfit that you really don't like anyway.

V. Furniture and Supplies

Again, it is likely that she, or her family and/or friends have already had all the essential furniture in place for the past six months - in what used to be your room. In general, it is likely that you will already have such things as a baby monitor, baby swing, bassinet, assortment of binkies and teething rings, bounce seat, changing table, diaper bag, diaper genie or diaper pail, some type of playpen, wipes, toiletries, and medical supplies. (If you don't know some of these terms, see Glossary of "What Words to Know.") Yes, it may seem like you are establishing a hospital-in-a-box. But a well-supplied home MASH unit is critical toward making the inconvenient as convenient as possible.

BREAST FEEDING

Question: *Is breast feeding that big of a deal?*

Answer: In the distant past, breast feeding was thought to be such a vile activity, that it was predominantly practiced by those of lower socioeconomic stature, while as those of higher socioeconomic stature refused to consider it.

Nowadays, the opposite is true.

The reason for the switch is because word has gotten out that breast feeding has many important potential benefits that include:

* Breast milk changes in composition to provide the exact right stuff, at the exact right time of day, for the exact right age of the child.

* Breast milk is easily digested.

* Breast milk is always available, as long as the mother is around. No heating or cooling required. And it can be pre-pumped to be given even if the mother is not around.

*Breast feeding helps the child and mother bond emotionally.

* Breast milk has antibodies that may help fight infection

in the newborn.

* Breast feeding may help prevent the development of allergies to proteins in cows' milk.

* Because breast milk has calories, breast feeding may make it easier for the mother to lose weight after delivery.

* Breast feeding may reduce the risk of breast and/or ovarian cancer in the mother.

* Breast feeding may improve tooth development in the child.

* Breast-fed children may have less risk of obesity when they grow older.

* Breast milk is free.

* Best of all, unless the milk has been pre-pumped and stored, breast feeding requires ***her*** to feed the baby.

You get to stay in bed.

Question: *How soon after the baby is born will it begin to breast-feed?*

Answer: This could happen as soon as the baby is born, but most likely will not occur until after the baby has been brought from the nursery to the mother's hospital room.

Question: *What problems might she have with breast feeding?*

Answer: The most common initial problem is that junior may need correct directions to the oasis. In fact, the nurse will likely spend a good bit of time describing all types of ways to manipulate the baby toward handling the whole breast nipple situation. And even if the baby is a quick learner, it may take some time for her breasts to provide enough milk for the child. During this time, formula supplements may be necessary.

The main symptom problem with breast feeding is that the nursing mothers' breasts can become very sore. And while ice packs would probably offer considerable relief, many opt for the more readily available bag of frozen vegetables, and use that as an ice pack.

The important thing to remember . . . and this cannot be stressed enough . . . ***leave the vegetables in the bag!***

Afterwards, one would suppose, it would be O.K. to complete the thawing of the vegetables for possible use later on, perhaps in a stir fry recipe.

Some women choose to collect breast milk with a breast pump, which is kind of like your old fish tank filter, only in reverse. The breast pump pumps the milk into a bottle that you can feed to the baby.

Question: *I am knowledgeable of the medical literature regarding the benefits of breast feeding. I think she needs to breast feed. She doesn't want to. What do I do?*

Answer: You may have the knowledge, but she has the breasts, buddy. You have just been trumped. The point is, if she is uncertain about the whole idea of beast feeding, listen to her concerns and try to help her make the decision. While almost all health professionals seem to be in favor of it, it is still a highly personal choice that each mother is entitled to make. Also keep in mind that many women decide before the baby is born that they are going to breast-feed, only to discover once the baby comes that they can't or have decided not to.

Question: *She really wants to breast feed, but her breasts aren't cooperating. She can't get any milk. Now she thinks that the kid is going to grow up sickly, and that she is not a good mother. What do I do?*

Answer: Many reasons exist why mothers can't, or shouldn't breast feed. And while as most experts believe that breast milk is best, the fact is, millions of babies have been successfully raised without breast milk.

And if she doesn't breast feed, then you will probably be asked to assist in the whole baby feeding situation. And, as hard as it may be to believe, you may find that feeding the baby from time-to-time is more fun than you thought it would be. In fact, you may become quite shocked about how well you adapt to this whole new father situation.

Question: *How long should she breast-feed?*

Answer: Most obstetricians and pediatricians recommend breast feeding last anywhere from six weeks to one year - a pretty wide leeway. Although yet to be proven, it is generally thought that all emotional and nutritional advantages have probably all been achieved by the end of a year.

Yes, some couples think breast feeding should be continued until the kid is four or more years' old. But aside from just being weird, there is always the matter of ***teeth***.

Ouch!

THE TIME FACTOR

Question: *We just don't have the time to handle this.*

CHAPTER 15: After the delivery

Before she delivered, we both worked. On weekends, I would get off at a reasonable hour. We would then get dressed, go to a movie, out to eat, and go to bed well after midnight. We would then get up the next morning somewhere around noon.

Now that she has delivered, I have to work overtime. When I get home, we have this new life that occupies our every minute. And because our baby gets up so early, we usually are up by five or six o'clock every morning.

How do we get our life back? How do we handle this?

Answer: You will soon surprise yourself. Because no matter how disorganized and inefficient you were before, you will be amazed how well you adapt to the whole new baby situation.

You will soon find that even if you arrive home from work on Friday after 8:00 P.M., you will still have time to play with the kid, spend some quality time with your computer and/or tools while she washes four loads of clothes and all the dishes, have a pizza delivered, eat the pizza while watching a taped TV program (that you recorded earlier because neither of you had time to watch it during the week), put the kid to bed, put both of you to bed, make love to your wife, talk about what you both are going to do in the morning, and be asleep by 11:00 P.M.

The point is, you just need to be aware of what to know after the whole delivery situation, and what to know ***after*** she's expecting.

AFTERWORD

It is our hope that this book will help expecting fathers understand their role, or lack of their role during the whole pregnancy situation.

For those wimp fathers who want to limit their participation to the barest minimum, we have tried to define the bare minimum they should know. (Hey, it's your prerogative Mr. Cro-Magnon.)

For those caring fathers who strive to do everything possible to make the whole pregnancy situation as pleasant as possible for her, we give helpful hints to enhance the chances that they can rightfully demand that she, and her family and friends recognize them as great fathers. (No one will, but they should get a good laugh out of it. After all, ***she's*** the one who is expecting!)

For all those fathers in between who are just trying to do the best they can, we describe how to know what is natural (but not normal), how to avoid being tagged with that ill-deserved "insensitive," and "selfish" label, how this is not a reasonable or perfect world, and how to know what lines that we have all heard enough to know that they are never to be taken seriously.

And finally, even though we detail how the best thing about pregnancy is that it only occurs in women, it is our hope that after reading this book, fathers will know what to know when ***she's*** expecting.

GLOSSARY OF TERMS

Entering the baby world can often be a confusing endeavor. At every turn, the new father can expect to be bombarded with terminology that may be as difficult as Sanskrit to decipher. This glossary of terms may help.

BABY MONITOR:
This is such an essential piece of equipment for parents that it staggers the mind to imagine how parents in previous generations got along without it. Basically, it allows those who are in one area of the house to hear, through the use of an audio monitoring system, what is going on with the baby in another area - usually the baby's room. A video version is also available for parents who are ultra compulsive, and who may not trust their babies near any cash. The main benefit of the baby monitor is to alert parents of the baby's activity. For example, in the frightening event that the baby makes noises in the middle of the night, then you or mom can jump up immediately and take action. On the other hand, in the frightening event that the baby doesn't make noises in the middle of the night, then you or mom can jump up immediately and take action. Having the comforting knowledge that you will be adequately warned by these two potentially dangerous situations allows you and her time to get that sleep you both so desperately need.

BABY SWING:
A BABY SWING is an extremely popular shower gift. These are

either electronic or crank-operated gadgets that will gently swing with a rocking motion that babies seem to enjoy. Best of all, it might put baby to sleep (or simply shut it up) when all else fails. And a baby swing in the house is sure a lot more convenient than bundling the baby up, and taking it for a ride in the car, just to make it sleep.

BASSINET:
This is a temporary, portable bed for the baby, that will allow you to put the child down to sleep in whatever room you wish. It is essentially a big basket with wheels. Most parents use the bassinet during the first few weeks after the baby is born, since the child may be too small for its crib. And as with virtually everything associated with children, bassinets can often be ornate and expensive, but they certainly don't need to be.

BINKY:
This is but one of many slang words for a pacifier, an item which may become an integral part of your child's early life. Your baby may or may not take to a pacifier, and there will probably be much discussion as to when it should and shouldn't be given, which may lead to head-knocking arguments involving you, your partner, the child's grandparents, your pediatrician, or all of these people. Although it may be hard to believe that a word like "Binky" could generate such turmoil, it will.

BLANKET SLEEPERS: Fuzzy pajamas.

BOOTIES:
Little socks. Not boots. Not shoes. So why aren't they called "SOCKIES?" We have no idea.

BOUNCE SEAT: A seat that bounces.

BURP PAD:
This is a pad that is placed on the shoulder of the person who is burping the baby. Its purpose is to protect the "burpee" from the toxic effects of regurgitated eats from the baby that is being burped.

CHANGING TABLE:
This piece of furniture serves as the area on which your child will have its diaper changed. The table may stand alone, or may be integrated with a cabinet which contains lotions, powders and other necessary diaper-related items. Most likely, other pieces of furniture will also assume the role of the "changing table," and include the couch, the bassinet, the crib, the bed, the kitchen table, and virtually anything and anywhere else involving a flat surface that the baby is willing to remain still for a few moments.

CRIB SHEETS:
These popular shower gifts are very small sheets for very small beds.

DIAPER BAG:
This item will become like an extra appendage to you and your partner. Diapers are but one of the multitude of articles which will be kept in the diaper bag. Bottles, wipes, pacifiers, toys, change of clothes and any other baby-related items will be transported in the diaper bag. It's kind of like a combination suitcase, and briefcase for babies.

DIAPER GENIE:
This is a technological, engineering marvel fresh from the computer age. It is a receptacle that allows dirty disposable diapers to be stuffed into a lined container, wherein the diapers are then wrapped and stored until the container is full. As advanced as this highly sanitary equipment is, it still requires that ***someone*** physically remove the string of sausage-linked, dirty disposable diapers when the DIAPER GENIE is full. Nevertheless, it is very convenient, and also reduces diaper-related odors in the baby's room. Don't ask how it works. It's a matter of national security.

DIAPER PAIL:
A DIAPER PAIL is an old-timey, no frills diaper container. It is to a DIAPER GENIE what an abacus is to a personal computer, or a vinyl LP is to a compact disc. It is essentially a can or bucket with a top, filled with diapers. If a cloth diaper service is used, it may be provided as part of the contractual package. In any event, scented diaper pail liners and a nearby can of air freshener are highly recommended accessories.

EXERSAUCER:
This is a stationary, circular device in which the baby occupies the center of a saucer. Not only is this generally safe physical exercise for a new being who, at times, may seem to come from a saucer, but learning how to move, bounce, and spin without actually going anywhere may become a good lesson in the corporate work environment.

FORMULA:
FORMULA is a primary source of food for many babies. It is designed to duplicate the nutrients found in breast milk. It is available in powder or liquid form, and it ain't cheap. There are lots of rules regarding the use of formula, which is all part of the big conspiracy. You will probably wind up purchasing formula at some point, even if your partner is breast feeding. WARNING: Do not drink the formula yourself, unless the need arises, and you are out of syrup of ipecac.

LAYETTE:
This is a fancy French word which supposedly means the baby's entire wardrobe, which will be stored and prominently displayed in a ***closette*** until the little rascal is born.

MOBILE:
A MOBILE is a controversial shower gift item which some consider to be a safety hazard. Your child will most likely enjoy having fun toys dangling over its crib or changing table, and they are often musical and will help to lull the baby to sleep. Two

important considerations include that, as the child gets older, it may pull the mobile down and get tangled or possibly choked by the strings. The second important consideration is that you may come to loath the accompanying repetitive baby tunes such as "Farmer in the Dell." (And what is a "dell" anyway. We don't know. But we do know you may soon have the desire to change the "Farmer in the Dell" into the "Farmer in the "Diaper Pell," as described before.)

NIGHTGOWNS: Baby bags with draw string bottoms.

NUK:
This is a brand name of a pacifier, and is often used in favor of "binky" or "paci." This is not to be confused with "Nanuk," which is a term referring to something up north, or in Canada. In other words, Nanuk of the North may use a Nuk, but a Nuk does not have to be used by a Nanuk.

OB/GYN DOCTORS:
OB/GYN doctors practice Obstetrics and Gynecology. "OB" stands for Obstetrician, which is Latin for midwife, or "she who stares or stands before childbirth." But since many of these doctors are men, and since men's ego is such that they would probably object to being called a "midwife doctor," the more sophisticated title of Obstetrician is preferred. "GYN" is Greek for woman. Therefore, a Gynecologist is a doctor that provides medical care to women. Because "GYN" doctors mainly focus on ***certain*** women problems, one could suppose it would be

better if these doctor's name themselves something clearer, such as the Ear, Nose and Throat doctors do. However, given the choice between learning the word Gynecologist, or referring to the doctor a Ovary, Uterus, and Vagina doctor, we think Gynecologist is just fine.

ONESIE:

A ONESIE is a clothing item that most babies will use quite often during their young lives. It is a one piece undergarment which snaps at the crotch and is worn under the baby's clothing, pajamas, or, in warmer areas, by itself. One would suppose that if it were to become ripped in half, it would become a "twosie." Onesies are underwear. Dressy onesies with legs and arms, and used as clothes during winter are known as STRETCHIES (see below). Dressy onesies without legs and arms, and used as clothes during summer are known as ROMPERS (see below).

PACI: See "binky" and "nuk."

PEDIATRICIAN:

It is important to determine who will manage your baby's medical care once its born. Your family doctor may your choice. Or you may want to find a baby doctor, known as a pediatrician. Either way, don't assume that the obstetrician will manage mom, ***and*** the baby. In many cases, you will want to meet with the pediatrician ***before*** delivery to arrange a plan ***at*** delivery. In making your choice, you will need to consider such things as the doctor's educational background, reputation, personality, philosophy, office hours, office location, call coverage, hospital privileges, and most of all, insurance participation.

PORT-A-CRIB:

Also known as a PLAYPEN, these are portable lodgings for your child. It is a baby mobile home. If you want to visit someone while you have the baby, you will need a place to put your baby down to sleep. Because these devices fold up, they can be taken with you. The only problem is that you may find them to be torture - to you, not the baby. Because unless you have a degree from MIT, putting up and breaking down one of these monsters would even present a challenge to "Scotty" from the Enterprise.

RECEIVING BLANKET:

The name makes little or no sense. But basically this is a small blanket in which you will swaddle your newborn baby. (Swaddle means strips of cloth used to wrap the baby). Although it gets rather confusing, the basic plan is this. First, the baby is changed by placing the dirty diaper in the DIAPER GEENIE or DIAPER PAIL (see above). The baby is then cleaned with a WIPE (see below), the diaper is replaced, and the baby is placed in a ONESIE (see above). Then it is wrapped like a fruit pastry in a RECEIVING BLANKET. And confusing as this may all be, it should be recognized that the wrapping of the RECEIVING BLANKET requires the working knowledge of Hebrew clothing techniques, and a level of dexterity that you will master about the same time the child is too big to benefit from your expertise.

RICE CEREAL:
This is a powdered cereal that sometimes is used in a very dilute mixture to the baby's bottle to fake the child out that its belly is fuller, so that you don't have to give the bottle so often. But because this is more controversial than extraterrestrials, you should get approval from the doctor first. But, in a more traditional sense, it may be added to formula, and given by spoon to the baby - representing the first type of "solid" food which your baby will likely take. It is good training for the mouth and tongue (as if your child more needs help in this area). Finally, it's taste is extremely bland, kind of like rice. Imagine that.

ROMPERS:
One piece, sleeveless or short sleeve, legless ONESIE (see above) that is used as clothing during summer.

SIPPY (OR SIP) CUP:
This is a lidded cup with a small spout that the baby will graduate to after drinking from a bottle or breast. The SIP CUP is filled with some type of liquid, and the baby is encouraged to suck from the spout. The theoretical benefit is that because the cup is covered with a lid, there is less chance of spillage than from a regular cup. However, if the baby simply turns it over, or uses it as a projectile, then the forces of gravity prevail, and the benefit is lost.

SNOWSUIT:
Otherwise known as a BUNTING BAG. These are essentially

sleeping bags with arms and a hood.

STRETCHY/SLEEPER:
One piece, long-sleeved, ONESIE (see above) with legs and feet coverings that are used as clothing during winter

TEETHING RING:
As the baby's teeth begin to form, it will need to chew on various items. Teething rings are often filled will a chillable gel which can be refrigerated, and will sooth the pain which sometimes accompanies teething. The gel looks tasty, but you should never try to eat it.

WIPES:
A pure stroke of genius. These little beauties will be used constantly, every day, until your baby is ready to enter college. A larger and softer version of the ever-popular "moist towelette," they are stored in plastic containers (keep the lid closed on the wipe container, or you'll wind up with a box of dry paper) and are used for wiping the baby's bottom, face, hands and any other contaminated body parts. You'll wonder what your life was like before you started using them.

WIPE WARMER:
Electric heating pads that wraps around the box of WIPES.

INDEX

Index

Index

Book References:

What to Expect When You're Expecting.
Eisenberg A, Murkoff HE, Hathaway SE. 1991 Workman Publishing Company
What to Expect The First Year
Eisenberg A, Murkoff HE, Hathaway SE. 1989 Workman Publishing Company

1997 World Wide Web References

Ask Campus Ecology
http://www.linkmag.com/Link/oct_nov_95/Environmental.html
At-home medical tests
http://www.mayo.ivi.com/ivi/mayo/9602/htm/home_pre.htm
Childbirth.Org
http://www.childbirth.org
Chinese Lunar Calendar
http://www.holodeck.com/pregnancy/chinese-cal.html
Embryo Development Overview
http://www.med.upenn.edu/embryo_project/embryo.html
Epidural - Frequently Asked Questions
http://www.fensende.com/Users/swnymph/Epidural.html#proc
Family.com (by Disney)
http://www.family.com
Finding Out the Sex of Your Baby FAQ
http://www.childbirth.org/articles/decide.html#how

Just for Fun - Will it be a boy or a girl
http://www.childbirth.org/articles/boyorgirl.html
La Leche League - The Advantages of Breast-feeding
http://lalecheleague.org/
ParenTalk Newsletter
http://www.tnpc.com/parentalk/index.html
ParenthoodWeb
http://www.parenthoodweb.com
Parenting Q & A
http://www.parenting-qa.com/
ParentSoup
http://www.parentsoup.com/
Pregnancy Links
http://www.atkinson.yorku.ca/~sowk/kjl/preglink.html
Pregnancy Signs
http://www.ausoft.com/pregnancy/
Usenet (Newsgroups)
alt.parenting and misc.kids
Zero to Three
http://www.zerotothree.org

1997 Phone References

Child Care Aware 800-424-2246
ChildHelp National Hotline 800-4-A-CHILD
Gerber Information Line 800-443-7237
Healthy Mothers and Babies 800-637-8444
National Mothers of Twins Club 800-243-2276
National Parent Information Network 800-583-4135
Parents Anonymous 909-621-6184
Single Parents Association 800-704-2102
Triplet Connection 209-474-0885

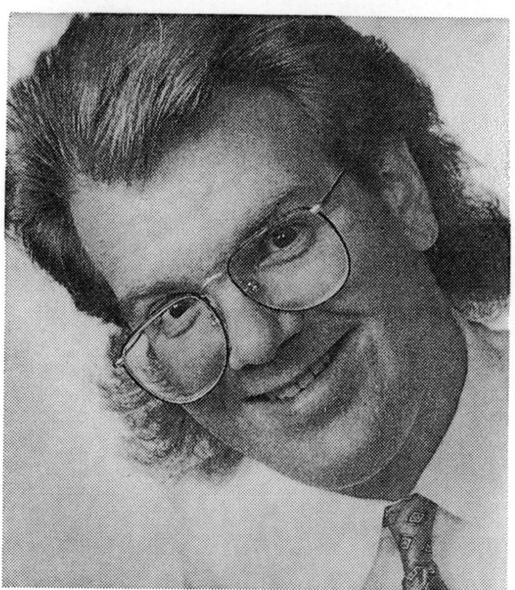

Mike Nilsson

Mike Nilsson has been a professional stand-up comedian since 1984. He has performed throughout the U.S., Canada and The Bahamas at comedy clubs, universities and corporate gatherings. He has performed with many of the biggest names in comedy, including Jay Leno, Jeff Foxworthy, Rita Rudner and Richard Jeni. He appeared in the 1985 film Summer Rental, directed by Carl Reiner and starring John Candy.

Mike lives in Louisville, Kentucky, wife his wife, Sheri, and his daughter, Grace.

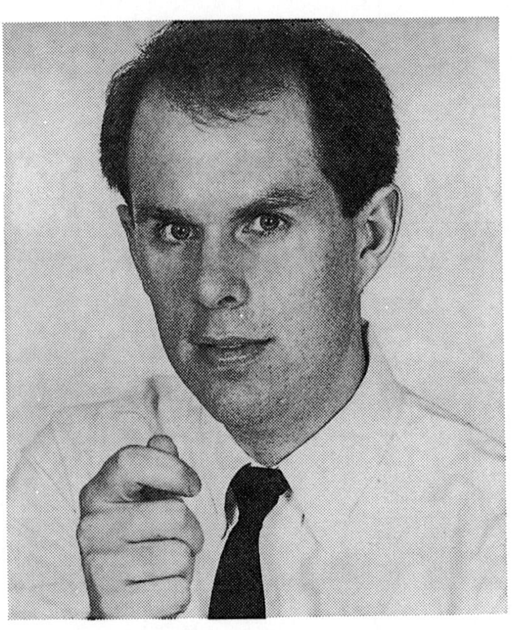

Harold Bays M.D., F.A.C.P.

"concerned about the health of the nation"

THE ONLY STAND-UP ENDOCRINOLOGIST IN THE WORLD

Health care issues have received much attention in the past several years. But one perspective has been ignored - a comic's perspective.

About the Authors

Dr. Harold Bays (the researcher) has been the featured speaker for numerous academic and medical programs. Dr. Bays ("The Only Stand-up Endocrinologist in the World") has performed at top comedy clubs around the country.

Since 1988, Dr. Bays has combined his medical knowledge with his comedy skills to raise tens of thousands of dollars to benefit patients with chronic diseases (such as cancer, arthritis and AIDS), the homeless, the United Negro College Fund, and other charities. He is probably best known as the featured comic of the "Stand Up Diabetes" program that has taken him around the nation to raise funds for the American Diabetes Association (ADA), and to increase awareness of this misunderstood disorder.

Dr. Bays first entered into comedy after being a professional musician (jazz, blues, and "60's" bands), busboy, dishwasher, cook, janitor, and clerk. His life's successes and failures have given him a unique political viewpoint on the issues of our times. For example, his concerns about the press have been detailed in his controversial book "The Perspective, Libel, and the Ten Rules of 90's Journalism" that has been featured on national cable, and talk radio.

On a professional level, Dr. Bays is the recipient of academic awards, is Board Certified in Internal Medicine and Endocrinology and Metabolism, is the Medical Director of a research center (conducting numerous phase II-IV clinical research trials in new and established cholesterol, diabetes, hypertension, and other metabolic treatments), is an

Endocrinologist in private practice, and has been elected as a Fellow of the American College of Physicians. He has published many worldwide medical articles on the evaluation and treatment of metabolic diseases, and has been a much sought after national lecturer to Universities and physician groups alike. In fact, he has given well over 150 lectures and media appearances regarding his expertise in various metabolic disorders such as cholesterol problems, diabetes mellitus treatments, high blood pressure drugs, thyroid disease, osteoporosis, and other such topics.

Finally, Dr. Bays has been "recognized with honor for his contributions to the medical profession and to the health and well being of the community at large" for his ongoing volunteer work with the homeless. He is also the distinguished, citywide winner of the second annual Louisville ADA "Kiss a Pig" fund raiser, and a recipient of a 1995 ADA "Spirit of Service Award."

Dr. Bays' viewpoints may be controversial, but his perspective is unique, genuine, and suggests you don't have to be from the east or west coast to have an opinion.

Dr. Bays lives in Louisville, Kentucky, wife his Dawn, and his son Jason.

About the Authors